LINDA WOLFE

An Imperfect Wardrobe

Ditch Monontonous Must-Have Lists, Stop Counting Your Clothes, and Curate A Wardrobe That Works For You

First edition

This book was professionally typeset on Reedsy.
Find out more at reedsy.com

Contents

Preface

THE PERFECT WARDROBE MYTH

Are you on the quest for a perfect wardrobe?

One where you effortlessly pull anything out of your closet and get dressed with no stress...

One that will help you realize your dreams of getting that job, landing that mate, and looking thinner, younger, and richer...

And one that ensures everything you buy works perfectly with everything you already own...

A perfectly streamlined closet that has the perfect pieces, allowing you to get dressed with perfect ease.

But instead, you find yourself fighting your closet every day because it's packed with unworn clothes that you can't seem to get rid of. You struggle to get dressed because you have no idea what's in there.

Then, to fix the situation, you go shopping, spending hundreds of dollars of hard-earned money on clothes you think will magically make your wishes come true. But, you never end up wearing most of these new pieces and you keep them until it's too late to return them. The clothes sit in your closet, unworn, causing you to feel guilty for buying them.

Does this sound familiar?

If so, you're probably wondering what you're doing wrong.

Why can't you have a perfect wardrobe?

You want to know the secret to getting this illusive perfect wardrobe that you keep reading about in articles like *How To Get The Perfect Wardrobe, The Essential Pieces Every Woman Needs,* and *Edit Your Closet In One Day.*

But what, exactly, does this mythical, perfect wardrobe look like?

Who defines wardrobe perfection?

And how do you get it?

According to most of the advice online, getting the perfect wardrobe is easy! Just fill your closet with an exact and minimal number of pieces that are on a generic master must-have list. **Some of the methods used to achieve said perfect wardrobe include:**

The Classic Method, a.k.a. Take everything out of your closet, throw it into a giant pile on the bed, and simply get rid of everything you don't wear. Those with a perfect wardrobe will not struggle and will easily remove all clothes, shoes, and accessories they never wear and will bag them up to donate.

Why this doesn't work: How will you suddenly be motivated and mentally prepared to spend your entire day purging over half of your wardrobe? You know that's what you're *supposed to do,* but parting with unworn clothes is hard and you need help and guidance.

The Get Back Your Money Method, a.k.a. Sell your cast-offs online and recoup your money. Apparently, those with a perfect wardrobe have lots of free time to take pictures of their clothes, and list them online.

Why this doesn't work: Unless you're selling designer pieces in really good condition, most of your clothes will not be worth much. And if they do sell it will be for a very small amount that might not be worth the time and effort. Plus, you have to make a special trip to the store to get the packing materials.

The Hanger Trick, a.k.a. Turn all your hangers backwards and flip them forward any time you wear something. Then, after an appropriate amount of time, get rid of everything that has the backward hanger because you didn't wear it.

Why this doesn't work: This does nothing to address the root causes of why you're not wearing those pieces. You know which clothes you do and do not wear without needing to turn hangers around. And a *perfect* wardrobe does not have hangers facing in different directions.

The Have "X" Number Of Clothes In Your Closet Method, a.k.a. Count all of your clothes and do not, I repeat, do not go over that number.

Why this doesn't work: I had to say "X" because the exact number of clothes you "should have" is different everywhere you look. Funny how the *perfect* number varies quite a bit from site to site. And I don't know about you, but I have no interest in counting and keeping track of the number of clothes I own. I have better things to do.

The One-In-One-Out Rule, a.k.a. Every time you buy something new you must get rid of something you already have.

Why this doesn't work: What if you've already streamlined your closet to *"perfection"* and don't want to get rid of anything else right now? And sometimes you want or need a new piece, like a bright blazer or a striped T-shirt, to liven up your wardrobe.

The Master Must-Have List, a.k.a. Make sure you have everything on this standardized must-have list, whether you work in an office, at home, or are retired.

Why this doesn't work: Generic must-have lists don't help because everyone has their own lifestyle needs and personal preferences. Not only this, but not all types of clothing work for everyone. Three pieces on every list I see that I don't own are the white, button-up blouse, the camel trench coat, and the sheath dress. I avoid button-up blouses because buttons always gap open across my large chest. Trench coats are too busy with all the flaps, buttons, cuffs, and belt. I invested in a sheath dress several years ago for "just in case," but I only wore it once and now it doesn't fit. You need to curate your own personalized wants and needs list because the *perfect* wardrobe looks different for everyone.

The Never Buy Anything Unless It Goes With "X" Other Pieces Method, a.k.a. When shopping, those with a *perfect* wardrobe make sure to never buy anything unless it goes with at least "X" other things in your closet. (There's that pesky "X" again). Oh, and wait a few days before committing to a purchase to ensure you really want it.

Why this doesn't work: When you shop with purpose and a plan just about everything in your closet should work with just about everything else. If you really like it, need it, and it's within your budget, then buy it now. Who wants to make another trip back to the store next week only to find your size or preferred shade is gone?

The Only Buy Complete Outfits Approach, a.k.a. Don't ever buy just one top, or one pair of pants, or one jacket. Those with a *perfect* wardrobe always buy a top, pants, and jacket at the same time to create a complete outfit.

Why this doesn't work: You can't always find what you need on a shopping trip. Sometimes it's necessary to go to a different store or a different mall. As I just mentioned, when your wardrobe is full of well-thought-out purchases, almost everything should work together rather than only working for a specific outfit.

I'm sure the people touting this advice have the best of intentions. And one or more of these methods may work for some people. However, the problem is most of it is redundant, outdated, limiting, restrictive, neurotic, unrealistic, and a hassle. There are too many rules that make the already stressful process of purging and shopping even more difficult.

So, forget about *perfection* and the idea of a *perfect* wardrobe. There are no wardrobe quick-fixes and no magic formulas. Besides, striving for perfection is simply unnecessary. The pursuit of perfection in any endeavor is a recipe for disaster. It sets up unrealistic expectations that are unattainable.

Instead, embrace the concept of an imperfect wardrobe.

What is an imperfect wardrobe?

An imperfect wardrobe is a flexible wardrobe that evolves according to your needs and lifestyle. It is a neutral approach to dressing that you personalize based on your specific wardrobe goals. An imperfect wardrobe has some mistaken purchases that need to go, and it has some category gaps that need to be filled, and that's okay. An imperfect wardrobe gets better slowly, over time. It requires ongoing evaluation, maintenance, care, and consideration to keep it functioning properly. An imperfect wardrobe is one that works for you and you alone.

What an imperfect wardrobe is not:

An imperfect wardrobe is not filled with a rigid number of clothes. It does have the right amount of clothes for your lifestyle needs and personal preferences.

An imperfect wardrobe does not have every item on someone else's must-have list. It does have the types of clothes, shoes, and accessories that you need for your lifestyle needs and personal preferences.

An imperfect wardrobe is not a carbon copy of anyone else, whether it be a famous person or a character in a movie or TV show. It is unique to you.

An imperfect wardrobe does not have an outfit for every possible scenario or occasion that could arise. It does have enough clothes, shoes, and accessories to comfortably get you through your daily activities. And it has several versatile pieces that can be dressed up or down for various situations by changing a few accessories.

An imperfect wardrobe is not filled with high-end designers, nor is it stuffed with inexpensive "finds." It is a balanced mix of price points.

An imperfect wardrobe takes more than one afternoon to edit. Getting rid of unworn clothes is an emotional experience that takes time. And it gets easier as you see the results.

And imperfect wardrobe has occasional mistakes. After all, you're human. When you do make a bad purchase, you return it, you learn from it, and you don't repeat it.

And an imperfect wardrobe is not static. It evolves over time with each new purchase and each round of editing, so it will never be perfect. And that's okay.

So, how will this book help you curate your imperfect wardrobe?

In **Part 1,** we'll examine **Why You Keep Clothes You Never Wear.** We'll tackle all those utterly lame excuses, crush those "until" thoughts, and figure out what you want and need from your wardrobe. Once you shift your mindset, you'll see why there's no reason to hold onto unworn clothes. You'll also think about what you want and need from your clothes going forward.

Then, in **Part 2,** you'll be ready to **Audit and Edit Your Wardrobe** *without taking everything out of your closet and throwing it on your bed.* You'll be working in batches, by category, so you can go at your own pace. We'll also analyze your closet setup to ensure you are maximizing your space. Once everything is organized and streamlined we'll discuss how to maintain order to ensure your wardrobe continues to work for you. You don't want to put in all this time and effort only to return to your old habits and old mindset.

In **Part 3**, we'll examine **Why You Buy Clothes You Never Wear** and what to do about it. By looking at your shopping style, you can pinpoint your purchasing triggers and wardrobe weaknesses. Plus, we'll discuss tricks and tactics retailers use to get you to pull out your wallet, the real cost of your clothes beyond the price on the tag, and how to find the best stores for you.

Lastly, in **Part 4,** we'll look at **Shopping Strategies**. You'll do pre-planning to determine what pieces are missing and create a strategy to acquire those items. We'll go over shopping trip tips for smarter shopping sessions, as well as discuss post-shopping evaluations. These are important, yet overlooked, parts of curating your imperfect wardrobe.

To ensure you get the most out of this process, use this book in conjunction with the free *An Imperfect Wardrobe Workbook*. It's jam-packed with all the printable worksheets and checklists you need to keep you focused and on track. **Download your free bonus *An Imperfect Wardrobe Workbook* at https://closetcures.com/an-imperfect-wa rdrobe-workbook/** And be sure to check out **ClosetCures.com** for even more useful information.

One final note: This book is not about getting results in one day, one week, or even one month. This is an ongoing process. Your imperfect wardrobe is an evolving thing. It isn't static. It needs attention and care.

You won't get rid of every piece of clothing, every pair of shoes, and every accessory that you never wear after reading this book. That's unrealistic. You did not accumulate all these clothes overnight. And you'll not be mentally prepared to part with every unworn piece the first time you edit your closet. And you'll still occasionally succumb to the lure of sales and clearance items. That's why you keep the receipts. Don't let this discourage you. It's perfectly normal when you have an imperfect wardrobe.

As you experience the bliss of a progressively streamlined and organized closet, you'll find that getting rid of unworn clothes gets easier. And, as you continue to refine your wants and needs, your shopping trips will be more productive and successful.

This is your journey to curating an imperfect wardrobe that you works for you.

Are you ready?

Then let's get started...

I

Why You Keep Clothes You Never Wear

An imperfect wardrobe will always have a few clothes, shoes, and accessories that you don't wear. But having too many unworn clothes creates chaos and confusion, making it more challenging to get dressed each day. Getting rid of excess pieces allows you to get dressed without the stress and reduces feelings of anxiety and guilt over wasted money and mistaken purchases.

However, the purging process is not easy. Before you start evaluating your clothes you need to get into a mindset that will set you up for success. Understanding why you're keeping clothes you never wear is the key to parting with them. This is a vial step that is often overlooked. To get into this mindset you're going to look at your clothes with an objective eye, and answer some questions to help you determine what you want from your wardrobe. You'll learn to turn negative thoughts into positive mantras, why more options are not necessarily better, and why most excuses are utterly lame. After completing part one you'll be mentally prepared to make the tough decisions during your wardrobe audit and edit. Download your free bonus An Imperfect Wardrobe Workbook at https://closetcures.com/an-imperfect-wardrobe-workbook/

1

What Kind Of Closet Do You Have?

Let's look at your closet as it is right now. Try to be objective and view it like it isn't your closet.

What do you see when you open the closet doors?

Is there a sea of bright prints and colors? Or lots of neutrals and a few muted shades?

What would you think if this wasn't your closet, but rather, a stranger's?

What would be your impression of that person?

Would you think they were highly organized and had great taste, or would you think they were confused and that their closet lacked any order or cohesiveness?

Below are several different kinds of closets. We'll discuss why they're causing a problem and what to do about it. Try to identify which imperfect closet you most identify with. Chances are, you're a combination of a few...

The Aspirational Closet

There are many clothes that you don't wear because they're not appropriate for your lifestyle. You have pieces that you would like to wear but they are too formal for your leisure activities or too casual for work. Or, you have a bunch of workout gear, but you never started working out.

The problem: You don't have enough of, or the appropriate clothes for, your current wants, needs, and lifestyle. Instead, you have too many pieces for your fantasy life.

The solution: Focus on the clothes you need for your daily life. If there's a new activity you want to try that requires specific types of clothes start with just one outfit. Make sure this will be a new normal activity, and then add additional pieces as needed.

The Multiple Sizes Closet

You have clothes in several different sizes because your weight fluctuates, or you never get rid of anything.

The problem: When you grab something, you don't know if it will fit or not. And if it's too tight, you instantly start to feel depressed or anxious. Garments that are too big are also problematic because they're not flattering and can make you look frumpy.

The solution: Only have clothes in your closet that are your current size. If your weight tends to fluctuate store select pieces in other sizes somewhere else. Just don't have a whole other wardrobe on standby.

The Mediocre Closet

Your clothes are okay. Nothing too exciting, bright, or bold. You tend to have multiples of many items most of which are basics.

The problem: Everything kind of looks the same. And you don't love any of it. Your wardrobe is not that interesting.

The solution: Make sure the core pieces you do have are in good condition and of high quality. Then work on injecting some color, pattern, and texture in small doses to bring more interest to your wardrobe. Try to identify which basic styles you're most attracted to. From here, you can try new colors, patterns, and a few trendy, non-basic updates every season.

The Confused Closet

Your closet is all over the place. There is no unifying theme or style. You have lots of price points, sizes, colors, and styles. You have both old and new pieces and everything in between.

The problem: Nothing works together. The colors clash and the styles are at odds. Half of the clothes don't fit properly.

The solution: Explore your personal style tendencies to identify the types of garments you like. Buy most of your clothes at just a few of your favorite retailers to get consistent fit, color coordination, and harmony.

The Dated Closet

You've had most of your clothes for a very long time because you never get rid of anything. You don't buy clothes very often. And when you do, they are the same style as what you already have.

The problem: Your garments may be in good condition, but they look dated and out of style. Or they're well-worn and are no longer crisp and fresh.

The solution: Plan to update the main pieces if you like the general style. But don't be afraid to try something new now and then. Spend less on trial pieces and invest more on updated versions of the basics you like.

The Trendy Closet

You only wear most items once or twice, for just one season. Your clothes are a wide variety of colors, styles, and prints.

The problem: You don't have enough core pieces or basics making it hard to put together outfits. Because trendy pieces become dated very quickly and you lack a solid stock of basics, you almost need a whole new wardrobe each season.

The solution: Work on creating a core of well-made basics that you'll have for a few years. Then add in a few trendy pieces that you like each season. This way, you'll still be current without needing to constantly update your entire wardrobe.

The Clearance Closet

Just about everything was bought on sale or clearance. You can't find anything that you paid full price for.

The problem: The colors are slightly off or unique, the fabrics are synthetic, the construction is not the best, and the styles look stale. You struggle to create outfits that work together.

The solution: Steer clear of the clearance section because it's too tempting for you. It is not a good deal at any price if you don't wear it. Spend that money on core pieces that you won't find on the "last chance" rack. Remember that high quality basics are always in style.

The Packed To The Brim Closet

You never get rid of anything. You've never attempted to purge or organize, and you truly have no idea what all is in there.

The problem: You can never find anything when you need it. And you know there are lots of clothes, shoes, and accessories you don't want and never wear but the thought of digging into your stuffed closet for a marathon purging session is just too overwhelming.

The solution: Break things down into manageable chunks. Only work on one category at a time. You don't have to tackle your entire closet in one day. But you'll be motivated to keep going once you see the positive results.

Which Closets Can You Relate To?

Do you have a closet packed to the brim with clearance items? Or a mediocre closet filled with multiple sizes? Perhaps you have an aspirational closet with multiple sizes that's packed to the brim.

Regardless of the *type* of closet you have, *the* solutions are all very similar. In fact, you could call it a road map for having a closet filled with clothes you wear.

You need a core of quality basics (whatever basic looks like for you) which you invest more on. Then, add in a few lower-priced trendy pieces each season to create new interest and remain current.

The quality neutrals will last for several years. This makes them worth the higher price tag, while the less expensive, trendier pieces will get lots of wear for that season. Because you didn't spend too much on the trendy clothes, you won't feel guilty parting with them when they fall out of fashion.

2

What Do You Want From Your Wardrobe?

Now that you've analyzed your closet like it belongs to a stranger, you may be itching to get in there and get to work. Before you do, you need to be clear about the results you are trying to achieve. It's important to conduct a self-analysis about your wants, your needs, and your attitude toward your clothes.

We're going to explore how you feel about your current wardrobe and uncover what you aspire to get from your clothes. The reason for doing this is because you need to know what's wrong before you can make it right.

This involves asking the *right* questions to get the *true answers* because I want you to really understand your feelings and attitude toward your clothes.

You need to ask many questions, not just the standard, "Do I like it, do I wear it, and does it fit?"

Below are a series of questions designed to make you really think about your wants, needs, personal style, and preferences. Answering these questions is so important because the answers will guide you toward crafting your personalized wardrobe.

Keep your answers simple, straightforward, and specific. You must narrow your focus, otherwise, you'll be all over the place. I've provided examples and guidance about the *types* of answers you should be giving. Of course, your answers will be specific to you and you alone.

Again, asking the right questions and providing the right types of responses will bring you the best results.

Use the worksheets from your free bonus *An Imperfect Wardrobe Workbook* to record your answers. Get your free workbook at https://closetcures.com/an-imperfect-wardrobe-workbook/

My three main goals for my wardrobe and the vibe I want to project are: (example)

1. To create more of an edgy rocker vibe that's laid back and casual
2. To stop buying pieces that are too boring and too classic because they don't truly fit my style
3. To create more interest with accessories

My three main goals for my wardrobe and the vibe I want to project are:

1. _____
2. _____
3. _____

How I will achieve these goals: (example)

1. Identify the types of pieces that will help me achieve the edgy

rocker vibe I'm going for
2. Find new brands and stores which carry merchandise that has a bit more variety
3. Start wearing more accessories

How I will achieve these goals:

1. _____
2. _____
3. _____

I want to avoid looking: (example)

1. Dumpy and frumpy
2. Feminine and girly
3. Uptight and overly formal

I want to avoid looking:

1. _____
2. _____
3. _____

I will avoid looking like these descriptions by staying away from: (example)

1. Oversized, baggy clothes in drab shades and plain, baggy chinos

2. Feminine and girly details like lace, ruffles, and pale pink
3. Uptight and overly formal features like button-up shirts, heels, tailored suit jackets, and trousers

I will avoid looking like these descriptions by staying away from:

1. _____
2. _____
3. _____

I hate shopping for: (example)

1. Pants, shorts, jeans – because finding bottoms that fit right is challenging
2. Bras - because there are so many styles and cuts I don't know where to start
3. Formal work clothes - because I prefer attire that is casual and laid-back

I hate shopping for:

1. _____
2. _____
3. _____

Unfortunately, these categories that you hate shopping for are likely the ones you'll need to spend the most time on *because* they're your biggest challenge areas. The things you hate shopping for require that you focus the entire shopping trip on just that category.

When you find pieces in your problem categories, like pants or bras, that fit you well and that you feel confident in, be sure to buy a few pairs in different colors. And remember the brand or store so you can revisit it the next time you need these items again.

I love shopping for: (example)

1. T-shirts
2. Jackets
3. Shoes

These are the pieces or categories that you're always drawn to and will undoubtedly have the most of in your closet because you love shopping for them.

But these are also the pieces that sidetrack you when you have every intention of looking for your problem categories like new bras.

For me, it's T-shirts, jackets, and shoes. I have all three in abundance, and in various incarnations and colors. It's great to have so many options and to enjoy certain pieces.

However, this often means other categories are lacking, like the aforementioned bottoms, because I hate shopping for pants and shorts.

I love shopping for:

1. _____
2. _____
3. _____

My three all-time favorite pieces are: (example)

1. Blue crinkled pigskin leather jacket - beautiful color and texture, unique, everyone complimented me on that jacket
2. Full-length black leather jacket - it was edgy and expensive which made me feel edgy and well dressed
3. Off-white lightweight cropped jacket with gold buttons - it could be casual or dressy depending on what I wore with it

These are pieces you've had that you absolutely loved! They can be pieces in your closet right now or from your past that you recall fondly. Why do you love them? What was it about them that you liked so much?

How did it make you feel when you were wearing them?

My three all-time favorite pieces are:

1. _____
2. _____
3. _____

Three celebrities whose style I admire are: (example)

1. I love Gwen Stefani with her many different looks even though I would never wear most of her wilder outfits. What I do like is that no matter what she's wearing, it always has an edgy rocker vibe because of how she combines pieces. Gwen wears lots of cargo pants, leather pants, jeans, boots, and tank tops. And she's never too revealing.
2. Angelia Jolie is another celebrity whose style I admire. Although

13

she is the opposite of Gwen in that she wears neutral, subdued shades, and lots of monochromatic ensembles. At the same time, she is bold and strong. She has a very classic style but adds some edge with pieces like black combat boots or leather pants. Angelia's accessories are typically minimal with simple jewelry. But she does carry an oversized luxury handbag. Frequent outfits include either long and loose pants, or tight leather pants, tanks or camisoles, and a light jacket or shawl. She always looks casual and comfortable without being sloppy or slovenly.

3. Cindy Crawford. Again, she has a casual yet pulled-together style. Cindy is typically seen wearing jeans, leather pants, tanks, T-shirts, light jackets, casual hair, great handbag, minimal jewelry, and oversized sunglasses. She usually has her shirts tucked in and wears a belt, which I never do, and she wears a lot of scarves which I also tend to avoid. But overall, I like her style.

The point is this: You can like someone's style, but you don't have to, or want to, copy it. Use their style as inspiration for your wardrobe. Look for the similarities in those whose styles you admire, and then take bits and pieces to emulate those qualities.

Even though all three women I mentioned are very tall with super long legs, and I'm only 5'4" with shorter, chunkier legs, I can still wear clean lines, monochromatic shades, and minimal accessories. And I can create interest and edge with rich textures and high-quality fabrics.

If you're not sure why you admire someone's style, type their name in online, click on the images tab, and look at the compilation of pictures. You'll see a pattern in the pieces they wear, the silhouettes they create, the colors they choose, and the vibe they project.

Three celebrities whose style I admire are:

1. _____
2. _____
3. _____

The three most important features that I want for my wardrobe are: (example)

1. Comfort
2. Edge
3. Quality

The three most important features that I want for my wardrobe are:

1. _____
2. _____
3. _____

When I think about my clothes the following thoughts come to mind: (example)

1. I wish I had some cooler pieces
2. I have a few pieces I really love and wear all the time, but the rest never gets worn
3. I have tons of casual clothes but nothing for when I want to step it up a notch

When I think about my clothes the following thoughts come to mind:

1. _____
2. _____
3. _____

The problems I typically encounter when getting dressed are? (example)

1. I'm always searching for something I know I have but can't find
2. I tend to get dressed quickly but never feel quite right. And then, halfway through the day, I catch a glimpse of myself and wonder what I was thinking?
3. I have a meltdown or anxiety attack every day as I try to assemble an outfit

The problems I typically encounter when getting dressed are?

1. _____
2. _____
3. _____

The negative mindset thought patterns I tend to have that are holding me back include? (examples)

1. I don't know how to put together outfits
2. I have no sense of style

3. Nothing ever fits me right

The negative mindset thought patterns I tend to have that are holding me back are?

1. _____
2. _____
3. _____

I'm ready to take back control of my closet and my wardrobe because: (examples)

1. I want to find items with ease
2. I want to feel confident and pulled together no matter what I'm doing
3. I'm ready to dress in my true style

I'm ready to take back control of my closet and my wardrobe because:

1. _____
2. _____
3. _____

*****

By completing this exercise you now have a better grasp of how

you do and do not want to look. You've explored your wardrobe strengths and weaknesses, and you've identified what's important to you when it comes to your clothes.

This knowledge will help you when we get to the auditing and editing section of this book. It will also help you to make smarter decisions when shopping.

But, this knowledge alone isn't enough to help you make difficult purging decisions about what stays and what goes. That's why we're going to examine your mindset to figure out why you're having trouble getting rid of clothes you don't wear. You'll learn how to identify and stop negative thoughts, and turn them into positive mindset mantras.

3

Mindset: Flip The Switch

When you are at war with your wardrobe you're likely engaged in a negative mindset filled with self-deprecating thoughts. You think you are the problem when the reality is you simply bought the wrong clothes for your shape, personal preferences, and lifestyle. The great news it that you can shift a negative mindset to a positive mindset. When you learn to do so, you'll experience a feeling of freedom and control that you didn't have before.

In this section, you're going to learn how to flip the switch on those destructive, negative thoughts and turn them into positive mantras. To do this, you must take control of your mind instead of letting your mind control you. This is the act of practicing mindfulness by shifting your mentality.

But, what is mindset and mindfulness?

Mindset is your collection of beliefs and thoughts that influence everything you do, from your choice of clothes and career, to your shopping patterns and behavior, to how you view yourself, others, and the world.

The **act of practicing mindfulness** is the determination to shift your thoughts to a positive mentality. It snaps you back to reality when those negative thoughts try to creep in.

Your mindset also impacts how you approach your wardrobe. When you have a pessimistic mindset, you blame yourself for unworn clothes instead of acknowledging that you simply made a purchasing mistake, and you can probably just return it. But, in your quest for the *perfect* wardrobe, nothing will ever be good enough.

Instead of feeling bad, retrain your brain to think in terms of what works for your *imperfect* wardrobe. Use any mistakes and struggles as a learning experience.

So, how do you get into this new mindset?

Step 1: Acknowledge that you're ready to adjust your mindset and start to flip the switch.

You must be ready to embrace the process. You must choose to be ready (i.e. get into a positive mindset) to change your way of thinking from destructive critiques and into positive thoughts.

Step 2: Identify your counter-mindsets or your negative fixed mindsets.

These are the negative, self-sabotaging thoughts and limiting beliefs that run through your head. Once you commit to having a realistic mindset regarding your clothes, you'll notice and become hyper-aware of your adverse thoughts.

Step 3: Stop negative thoughts immediately and turn them into positive mindset mantras.

As soon as you realize that you're telling yourself unfavorable and unrealistic things, flip those unfavorable and unrealistic thoughts into positive, realistic thoughts. When you find you're having these recurring, detrimental points of view, you can shift your thinking. And you can use these mindset tools in everything you do, not just with your wardrobe.

Below are some typical examples of negative thoughts and suggestions on how to shift your thinking to flip them into positive affirmations.

Negative Mindset Example: I'll never have an organized closet because it's too small, so what's the point?

Flip It: I'll get rid of everything that I don't wear. Then, I'll determine what types of storage solutions I can use to maximize the space I have.

Negative Mindset Example: I've tried many times to get rid of the clothes, shoes, and accessories I don't wear, but I still have way too many unworn items, so why bother?

Flip It: I'm finally ready to tackle my wardrobe thanks to my new mindset. My goal is to only have clothes I like and wear in my closet. I realize this is an ongoing process. I won't have a fully streamlined closet after just one attempt, but it will get better over time.

Negative Mindset Example: I can never find any clothes that I really like or that fit me right.

Flip It: I'll keep searching for stores that carry clothes that work for my personal style, lifestyle, and that fit my wants and needs. It's the stores and the clothes that are the problem, not my body.

Negative Mindset Mantra: I can't afford to buy clothes that I love. They often cost more than I wanted to spend, and I'll feel guilty for buying them.

Flip It: I'll focus on fit, how it makes me feel, and how often I will wear it, rather than the price tag. It makes sense to spend more on a few pieces that I'll love instead of spending less on clothes I might never wear and don't even like.

Negative Mindset Mantra: I can't do *insert activity here (such as go to the gym, go dancing)* because I don't have anything to wear.
Flip It: I'll buy clothes for the activities I like to do regularly.

Part of a negative mindset is telling yourself that you can't do something or buy something *until* everything is *perfect*. These are what I like to call **"until" thoughts.**

You know what I'm talking about...

Those thoughts you tell yourself that cause you to put off making wardrobe improvements **until** something happens such as:

*I can't buy new clothes **until** I lose weight, **until** I get that raise or promotion, or **until** my kids move out and start paying their own way.*

But putting things off until everything is *perfect* is a recipe for stagnation because nothing will ever be *perfect*. No situation is ever *perfect*.

Will you ever be 100% happy with your weight?

Will you ever be 100% happy with a job?

And do you really want to wait years for your kids to grow up to focus on your appearance?

These are simply ways of stalling. And they are counterproductive.

That's why you must crush these *"until"* thoughts by getting into the habit of taking action right now regardless of your circumstances.

Here are just a few examples of how you might adjust your mindset:

- Buying fun, stylish new workout clothes will encourage you to hit the gym. Compare that to wearing your old, baggy sweatpants and oversized T-shirt to work out. When you look and feel frumpy you'll feel self-conscious while exercising.

- Investing in better quality work clothes that you infuse with elements of your personal style can help you enjoy work a bit more. This can translate into a positive attitude that might result in better performance reviews to help you get a promotion or a raise. However, continuing to wear your dated and fading work clothes will cause you to fret about your appearance all day. This can make you grumpy and insecure, taking the focus away from your work.

- Paying attention to your appearance today and every day is not only important for your own self-esteem but for how your kids see you. You don't want them to be embarrassed to be seen with you because of your ill-fitting outfit and dated wardrobe.

When you catch yourself indulging in any form of negative mindset thoughts, stop them immediately and turn them into new mindset mantras. Realize that it takes time to get into the habit of adopting a positive mindset, so keep at it.

A good way to learn to adjust your thinking is to write down pessimistic thoughts when they pop into your head. Once you see the adverse thoughts in black and white, I want you to think about what you would tell someone else who said these things about themselves.

What would you tell your friend, sister, or daughter who said they are too fat to look good in blue jeans? You would tell them their weight is not the problem. They simply haven't found the best jeans and brand for their body.

Or if they said nothing ever looks good on them? You would tell them it isn't them, it's the clothes. And they just need to keep searching until they find the brands and styles that work for them.

This is flipping negative thoughts into a positive, optimistic mindset. When you flip negative thoughts, you must then create new concepts that encourage you to keep going.

Changing your mindset around your appearance and wardrobe does take some time and effort. But the more you practice **flipping the switch**, the easier it gets. Pretty soon, new habits and thought patterns will become automatic.

Taking small, steady steps toward change is more effective than having a one-day marathon closet clean out or going on a major shopping trip.

As you get rid of unworn clothes you'll start to see space in your closet which cuts down on the visual clutter. You'll be motivated to keep going. This is what many people refer to as the snowball effect.

But it's also important to realize that you will have setbacks, and that's okay.

There will be days when you hate everything in your closet, or when you get frustrated trying on clothes at the store. But don't use these setbacks as an excuse to just give up!

Rather, look at them as a learning experience.

Will you make a bad purchase now and then?

Of course. That's why you keep the receipts. And that's why stores have generous return policies.

Changing your mindset about your wardrobe and appearance means spelling out what you want out of life: your goals, the type of job you desire, and your lifestyle.

Without clear direction, how will you know where to go?

You must align your wardrobe with your goals, your body, and your lifestyle. Then, you can start working toward these goals.

List three negative thoughts that you've told yourself about your clothes. Then examine the real reason. (example)

Thought: I always look out of place at work because my clothes are too casual.

Reason: Maybe I'm not buying the appropriate clothes because I'm in the wrong career and the types of clothes I'm required to wear make me feel awkward. I have an office desk job with a semi-formal dress code, but would prefer a career where I could be more active and that comes with a more relaxed dress code.

Thought: I can't find pants that fit me right because of my short legs and big thighs.

Reason: I haven't found the right brand yet for my body type. As a result, I'm buying the wrong cuts and styles. I just have to keep looking until I find the best brands, cuts and styles for my particular shape.

Thought: My outfits are boring and uninspiring.

Reason: I keep buying the same types of clothes at the same stores. I'm going to try shopping at some different stores that have new styles, colors, textures, and accessories.

When you stare at your wardrobe, lamenting about how you don't like most of it, what's going through your mind? Most of the time, your negative thoughts are not even about your clothes. They're about issues like your weight, your job, or anxiety about money.

List three negative thoughts that you can think of that you've told yourself about your clothes. Then examine the real reason.

Thought:_____

    Reason:_____

Thought:_____

    Reason:_____

Thought:_____

Reason:_____

*****

List of Steps To Adopt A Positive Mindset:
- Be ready to change
- Be aware of negative thoughts
- Flip those negative thoughts into positive mantras
- Crush those "until" thoughts
- Take the necessary steps
- Start slow and small
- Realize there will be mistakes, setbacks & stumbling blocks
- Learn from these challenges
- Keep going

Along with a positive mindset is the practice of taking action. And the time to start is now.

Right now.

No more *until* thoughts and no more excuses.

4

Misleading Mindset: More Options Are Better

Perhaps you're of the mindset that having more clothes gives you more options.

While it's certainly true that having ten blazers to choose from as opposed to five blazers definitely provides more options, the problem is *with* those options.

More options doesn't necessarily equal a better selection.

More options doesn't necessarily equate to liking those items.

And more options doesn't automatically translate into a wardrobe that's flattering and that fits properly.

Plus, you can only wear one outfit at a time and there are only so many days in a season.

When you only wear a small percentage of your clothes, the rest sit unworn in your closet. They take up valuable real estate, creating chaos and confusion when you get dressed.

Bottom line: More is just more!

More time wasted digging through piles of clothes and squeezing between hangers…

More money spent on clothes, shoes, and accessories you're not wearing...

More stress trying to find pieces that fit right and look good...

More visual clutter and chaos which translates into you feeling anxious and out of control.

So, are you picking up that I don't think more clothes, shoes, and accessories are the answer to getting a wardrobe filled with pieces you like and wear?

As I mentioned in the beginning, I'm not a fan of counting clothes, creating a minimalist wardrobe, or systems like the one-in-one-out method. However, having a closet stuffed with all sorts of tops, bottoms, shoes, and accessories is not the answer either.

The goal for your perfectly imperfect wardrobe is to have a closet filled with pieces that you actually like and actually wear. Everything else is just a distraction.

It's ultimately up to you to decide how many clothes you'll have in your closet. There is no magic one-size-fits-all number.

If you like having more choices and you regularly wear all your clothes, shoes, and accessories, then you may be happy with more clothes than someone else might feel they need. The key to how many clothes you have or need is based on your lifestyle, your personal preferences, and the size of your closet.

5

No More Utterly Lame Excuses

Parting with clothes you never wear and often don't even like should be easy.

You know you should get rid of everything that's too big or too small...

You know that you're supposed to get rid of all the clothes, shoes, and accessories that you don't wear...

And you're tired of dealing with your stuffed closet...

So why are you still struggling to get your closet under control? Why can't you simply get these pieces out of your closet and out of your life?

Because you're letting your mind get in the way by trying to rationalize why you need to keep something. This rationale also comes with a lot of emotions around issues like how much you paid, your plans to lose weight, and how you got the item in the first place.

When you have guilt about unworn clothes, shoes, and accessories **the worst thing you can do** is leave them in your closet as a constant reminder of wasted money, goals not yet reached, or guilt for not wearing a gift. These unworn items are controlling your thoughts.

Why do you want to feel bad every time you open your closet doors?

The best thing to do is get them out of your closet so you can focus on the clothes that you do enjoy wearing. Once you free yourself from these unworn items you'll feel liberated and in control of your wardrobe. So, how do you do this?

To successfully streamline your closet, you must get into the mindset that you're no longer going to keep things you don't wear regardless of money spent, unreached goals, or how you acquired the pieces. Getting into this mindset involves addressing the issues that are creating this struggle to part with inanimate objects. **Basically, you need to realize when you're simply making an utterly lame excuse for not getting rid of something.**

What are utterly lame excuses?

They are baseless stories you tell yourself to justifying keeping clothes, shoes, and accessories that you never wear, and often, don't even like. Making things even harder, many of the utterly lame excuses overlap.

For example, you may feel guilt due to cost or the condition of an item. You can't possibly get rid of that beautiful wool coat because you paid a lot for it, and it's still in great condition.

There's no way you can get rid of that hideous plaid sweater your grandmother gave you five years ago. It reminds you of her, and she would be hurt if she knew that you just threw it out.

And you might need that suit for a job interview someday, even though the shoulder pads instantly date the outfit, and the pants are a little snug.

How many times have you used one of the following utterly lame excuses for keeping clothes you don't wear and often, don't even like?

- I paid good money for it
- I can't just throw it out
- I'm afraid I won't have anything left
- It might come back in style

- I'm going to lose the weight
- But it still has the tags on
- I might need these clothes someday if I go back to work
- I love it even though it's worn out
- It was a gift
- It brings back good memories
- It's my wardrobe weakness
- But I plan on wearing it someday
- I better keep it just in case
- I'll wear it once I get the right pieces to go with it

Which of these utterly lame excuses sounds all too familiar?

Maybe you have some excuses that aren't even on this list.

Whatever your excuse, the key to overcoming it is recognizing and acknowledging it, so when it starts to creep into your head you can flip the switch and replace it with a new mindset mantra.

Let's look a little closer at this list of utterly lame excuses to see the common rational people tell themselves for why they must keep something. We'll see why these excuses are no good and learn how to get into the mindset that these pieces are not contributing to the functionality of your wardrobe, and therefore, must go.

Utterly Lame Excuses Due To Cost Or Waste

Cost / Money Spent

Rationale: *I paid a lot for that. I'm not going to just give it away or throw it out!*

Reality: *The money is long-gone, whether you keep it in your closet taking up space and making you feel guilty every time you see it, or whether you get rid of it.*

I get it! You work hard for your money. And you feel guilty for spending that money on garments you're not wearing.

But the money is gone. And keeping clothes you never wear just because you spent good money on them doesn't bring that money back. This is also known as sunk costs.

Accept that these are sunk costs, learn from these mistaken purchases, and move on to enjoy the clothes you do have and like. And vow to make smarter purchases the next time you go shopping.

As I mentioned earlier, you can try to sell the clothes you're getting rid of, but the process can be very time consuming. And unless the piece is in perfect condition and a designer brand you won't recoup anything near the original price you paid. If it doesn't sell you still have to get rid of it.

Scarcity Issues

Rationale: *We didn't have lots of spare cash to spend on clothing when I was growing up. We never got rid of anything even if we never wore it.*

Reality: *If you're not wearing something then it is just clutter. Rather than being a source of comfort and security, these unworn clothes are actually causing anxiety and confusion when you try to get dressed.*

Some people take comfort from having lots of stuff around them. It makes them feel safe and prepared, especially if money was, or still is, tight.

But getting these unworn pieces out of your closet once and for all will be like a weight lifted from your chest. You won't be confronted daily with your mistaken purchases.

If you do still struggle with finances or don't have a lot of spare cash for clothes, that's even more reason to think twice about any potential clothing purchases. Be sure to shop with a plan. Only buy what you really want and need. Then, enjoy wearing those pieces. When you don't have a closet full of bad purchases, you don't have to struggle with purging.

Fear Of Regret

Rationale: *If I get rid of too much, there won't be anything left! And what if I need it?*

Reality: *You will have lots of garments left and they will be the ones you like and wear. And if you haven't needed it this whole time, you won't even miss it.*

If you feel like you have nothing to wear, then don't be afraid to get rid of stuff. You're not wearing it now and never will.

What's the worst thing that can happen if you do get rid of those three pairs of heels that you haven't worn in years? Do you have at least one neutral pair left? Do you even wear heels?

Once you get unworn pieces out of your closet, you'll forget all about them, whereas, seeing them every day is a constant reminder of wasted money.

It Might Come Back In Style

Rationale: *Since it's still in good condition, I better keep it in case it comes back in style.*

Reality: *Did you wear it when it was in style? Probably not, since it's still in good condition.*

Even if a style "comes back" your garment will still look dated. That's because nothing comes back in the exact original form. It will be a slightly different cut, color, fabric, or length.

Your goal is to have a closet filled with clothes that are in style right now.

Utterly Lame Excuses Due To Weight

Plan / Hope To Lose Weight

Rationale: *This will fit me again when I lose some weight.*

Reality: *Did you wear it when it did fit? Or did you buy it for your future, slimmer self as motivation?*

If you rarely wore it when it did fit, will you really want to wear it again after your weight loss?

Many people try to use their clothes as a motivator to lose weight. But the opposite happens.

Instead, they make you feel like a failure...

Like you'll never be your ideal weight...

Ditch those clothes that make you feel bad every time you see them. Replace them with some fun, new workout clothes to inspire you to reach your weight goals.

Utterly Lame Excuses Due To Condition: Good and Bad

The Price Tag Is Still On

Rationale: *It's brand new and still has the tags attached.*

Reality: *You've never worn it. That's why the tags are still attached.*

Determine whether or not you actually like the piece.

If so, wear it. Now.

If not, get rid of it. If you bought the item recently and can return it, do so. Even if you can't get cash back, you may get store credit. Otherwise, get rid of it.

Seeing brand new and unworn items hanging in your closet only brings up feelings of guilt associated with cost and bad decisions. Again, once you get rid of them, you'll forget all about them.

Good Work Clothes From A Former Job

Rationale: *If I return to work, I'll need these business clothes again.*

Reality: *Are you planning to return to work at a job that requires this dress code any time soon? If not, get rid of these clothes. If so, do you love the* *clothes and are they flattering? If not, then out they go.*

When you're starting a new job or returning to work after time off you'll want some fresh, current clothes. This will help you look and feel confident, so you can focus on your job instead of worrying about how you look.

You Really Used To Like It and Wore It Often

Rationale: *I love this piece, but it's starting to look unpresentable.*

Reality: *You shouldn't have any guilt about getting rid of clothes that you wore so much that they got worn out. They had a good run. And you got your money's worth. So, say goodbye and move on.*

When clothes start to lose their shape, fade, or shrink but you love them, it can be hard to say goodbye. But if they aren't looking so good then they need to go.

Refresh your wardrobe with a similar replacement. Check out the same store or brand for an update.

Utterly Lame Excuses Due To Guilt / Sentimental

It Was A Gift

Rationale: *I should be thankful that someone felt so much for me that they gave me a gift. It would be rude to get rid of it (even though I really don't like it and probably won't ever wear it).*

Reality: *But you don't like it, it's not your style, it's a terrible color, and you'll never wear it.*

It helps me to think about things I've given to other people that I never see them using or wearing. Do your friends and relatives love, use, and wear everything you buy them? Plus, I don't really remember anything I got as presents last year or several years ago, do you? Chances are, neither will your gift giver.

To prevent future bad gifts, you can tell the gift giver what you do want and do like. Or, ask them to stop buying you clothes because you really like to try clothes on to ensure they fit.

Sometimes, though, you just need to say thank you to your gift giver. Then, get rid of it and move on.

Sentimental Items

Rationale: *I could never part with this. I was wearing it when...*
Reality: *This one is easy. Get it out of your closet and put it in a keepsake box.*

Just don't cling to every little thing or your keepsake box will quickly overflow. Take pictures of the least sentimental pieces and then let them go.

Wardrobe Weaknesses

Rationale: *You find a piece you love, so you buy it in every color offered.*
Reality: *If you truly love the style and it fits great, it's smart to stock up. Be careful not to stock up so much in the same style that you sacrifice buying other things you also need.*

When you love a style or type of garment you tend to have several versions. This is perfectly fine if you wear all of them. Otherwise, weed out the ones that you never wear.

Utterly Lame Excuses Due To Being Prepared

It Was On A "Must-Have" List

Rationale: *If the "expert" says I must have it, then I guess I must.*
Reality: *Create a personalized list of "must-haves" based on your lifestyle, wants, needs, and your personal style.*

Must-have lists are very subjective. And they are certainly not one-size-fits-all, as they might not pertain to your particular lifestyle, career, wants, needs, and preferences.

This is the danger of so-called "must-have" lists. When you buy something someone you've never met tells you to buy, it probably won't work for you. I've fallen victim to these lists, as I'm sure many of you have, as well.

Ignore master "must-have" lists and get rid of anything that's not on your personal must-have list.

But I Plan On Wearing It One Of These Days

Rationale: *I'm going to wear it. The situation just hasn't presented itself yet.*

Reality: *If you're not wearing it for your current lifestyle, then you likely never will.*

When you've had clothes for several years that you think you like but have yet to wear, then wear them this week. If you don't, get rid of them.

And if you attempt to wear them but then take them off before leaving the house because they didn't fit right or feel right, get those pieces out of your closet and get rid of them.

Just In Case...

Rationale: *But what if an unexpected situation comes up that I need it for? Or, this dress will be perfect if I get invited to a wedding this year.*

Reality: *When is the last time you had to go somewhere at the last minute that required clothes you didn't have? You probably can't think of one because you either had something to wear that would be just fine for this one last minute occasion or you knew about the event well in advance and had time to shop for an appropriate outfit, like for a wedding.*

It's good to be prepared for various activities and situations that might come up. But you don't need to have something for every single thing that could possibly ever happen. And again, if such a situation arises, will the item you bought five years ago still fit and look current, or would you be better off buying something new?

Instead of having pieces that only work for one occasion, try to have more versatile pieces that can be dressed up or down with different accessories, by throwing on a jacket, or by adding a different pair of shoes.

I Just Need To Find The Right Piece To Go With It

Rationale: *I'll wear it as soon as I find the right piece to coordinate with it.*

Reality: *How unique is this piece that you can't find anything to wear with it?*

If you're on the hunt for a missing piece then give yourself a deadline. If you don't make an effort to look for it or you can't find it, then it needs to go.

On the other hand, it might not be worth the time and effort to search for this elusive piece that will make this wearable. You might be better off letting it go.

Don't buy pieces that require you to buy other special pieces to go with it. Your goal is to assemble a wardrobe that's cohesive, works for your lifestyle and personal preferences, and easily mixes and matches.

*****

Don't let these utterly lame excuses for keeping clothes you never wear stop you from curating an *imperfect* wardrobe that works for you.

When purging it's all too easy to focus on the negative aspects of the process.

Instead, focus on the positive results.

Think about what you'll gain by getting these unworn clothes, shoes, and accessories out of your closet and life. Once they're gone, you'll forget all about them. Focus on how much easier it will be to select clothes you actually like from your streamlined closet.

Why You Keep Clothes You Never Wear Summary

You've looked at your closet and your clothes with an objective eye. You've thought about how you want to look and feel, as well as considered the vibe you want your outfits to give off.

You've realized that you must adjust your mindset regarding your clothes and immediately flip the switch on any negative thoughts that creep into your head.

You've learned to stop "until" thoughts in their tracks and will instead focus on the present.

You now know why having more options is not necessarily better.

And you've seen the list of utterly lame excuses for keeping clothes you never wear, and you understand why they're utterly lame.

Now, you're mentally prepared to face these issues head on as you do your wardrobe evaluation.

With this new mindset, group of goals, and determination to finally get your chaotic closet organized and under control, you're ready for Part 2: Auditing and Editing.

As you go through your clothes, shoes, and accessories during your wardrobe audit and edit, keep your overall goals in mind.

My wardrobe goals are (example): To reduce stress, overwhelm and chaos.

I will achieve these goals by: Clearing out unworn items that make me feel bad about myself when I see them, by getting rid of clothes that don't fit into the vibe I'm going for, and by moving past the issue of money spent.

My wardrobe goals are:_____

   I will achieve these goals by:_____

If you still insist on keeping a piece after seeing the reality of your rationale, then I present you with this challenge:

Wear it this week. Period.

If you just can't bring yourself to wear it then get rid of it.

If you do wear it, how did you feel with it on? Were you uncomfortable? Self-conscious? If so, it should go.

Don't make any excuses.

GET RID OF IT!

II

WARDROBE AUDIT AND EDIT

The time has finally come to start the wardrobe auditing and editing process.
With your new, positive mindset, you have the tools in place to successfully purge the clothes, shoes, and accessories that you don't wear.
As you go through your wardrobe, continue to remind yourself that the clothes themselves are not important.
Remember that any money spent is long gone.
And you're ready to make your life easier by reducing the stress that comes with an overstuffed closet.
Refer back to the list of Utterly Lame Excuses For Keeping Clothes You Never Wear and the No More Excuses List when you have trouble getting rid of pieces.
Use the Clothing Analysis Flow Chart to keep you on track and help you decide what goes. Consult the list of Fit Checks to remind you of any fit issues that you may have overlooked. And keep your wardrobe goals in mind. Ask yourself if each piece is in keeping with these goals. If not, out it goes! If your haven't already done so, download your free An Imperfect Wardrobe Workbook at
https://closetcures.com/an-imperfect-wardrobe-workbook/

6

Merchandise Your Clothes

There's one more step I want you to do *before* you start the audit and edit process and that is to merchandise your hanging clothes. **Merchandising your clothes** simply means that you're going to group similar items together by category and color.

The task of merchandising your hanging pieces can be done quickly and without creating a messy pile of clothes. Therefore, don't worry about merchandising clothes, shoes, and accessories that are on shelves or in drawers yet. Just focus on your hanging rack or racks.

Once your closet is merchandised you'll know right where to look to find something. Grouping items by type also enables you to see which styles, colors or categories you have in abundance and which are limited or lacking.

But don't start analyzing pieces yet. That will slow you down and impede your progress. Simply focus on categorizing and colorizing.

Now, go to your closet and open those doors.

You're going to quickly group all like items together on the hanging rod or rods. Depending on your closet setup you may have just one hanging rod, or several. Either way, just focus on your hanging clothes for now.

Put all the T-shirts, pants, dresses, button-up shirts, etc. together. Whatever categories of clothing you have, group them together within the closet. If you have specific clothes just for work or some other activity, arrange all of those in one section.

You may need to remove a handful of items to create the space to work *within the closet,* especially if it is truly stuffed. Just don't take your entire closet apart. Again, don't worry about the floor or shelf for now, as they require extra attention.

Some of you may already have your closet merchandised. If so, skim through to make sure nothing is out of place.

As you're progressing, within each category, start to group colors together from light to dark using the classic **Roy G. Biv method:**

- Red
- Orange
- Yellow
- Green
- Blue
- Indigo
- Violet

Neutral shades can all be grouped together and stationed either before the reds or after the violets. Or, the other option for neutrals is to put the lighter neutrals at the beginning (before the reds) and the darker neutrals at the end (after the violets).

Neutral shades include:

- White
- Gray
- Brown

- Navy
- Black

As for **prints and patterns,** they can go in one group next to the neutrals, or they can be split up and added to the color grouping that is most dominant in the print or pattern.

That's it. The hanging rod or rods are now arranged by category and color. You can quickly see each type of clothing, the assortment of shades, and how many pieces there are. This step alone makes getting dressed less stressful.

7

Analyze Your Clothes

Now that you have your hanging clothes grouped by category and color, it's time to start the evaluation.

Rather than removing everything from your closet and creating a massive pile on your bed, you'll remove and work on just one category at a time. This prevents becoming overwhelmed, keeps you focused, and provides stopping points to take a break or come back the next day.

It's up to you to decide if you want to tackle the entire closet in one day. Or, if you'll do half today and half tomorrow...

Maybe you'll work on it over the course of the week...

Just get started.

We'll begin with the newly merchandised hanging rod or hanging rods, and then move on to the shelves. Next, we'll tackle the floor. Lastly, we'll analyze any clothes, shoes or accessories that you have in dressers, nightstands, or any other furniture pieces like an armoire.

For those of you who have clothes in rooms and closets other than your main bedroom closet, analyze those last. As you go through each category, it's important to keep in mind that you're focusing on fit, whether or not you like each piece, and whether or not you ever wear it.

Don't get hung up on what pieces you may be missing. We'll delve into what you want and need, as well as how to curate your *imperfect* wardrobe, in Part 4. For now, the focus is on your current wardrobe and whether each piece should stay or go.

The Hanging Rack

We'll begin the wardrobe audit and edit by tackling the clothes on the newly merchandised hanging rod or rods.

Remove the first category from the closet. Let's use T-shirts as our example category. Put those on your bed, a stool, or portable hanging rack.

The idea is to see the volume of pieces you have in that category, as well as the varying styles and colors. You want to be looking for both similarities and differences between each piece within this category.

Take note of details like:

- the type of neckline (crew, v, u, scoop, square)
- the type of sleeve (tight, loose, or somewhere in-between)
- sleeve length (long, elbow, short, cap, sleeveless)
- length (where the hem hits on your body)
- fit (oversized, form-fitting, or somewhere in-between)
- fabric (100% cotton, a blend, pure synthetic)
- color (shade and intensity)
- pattern (if not a solid)

As you analyze the T-shirt category, you may be surprised to see you have five red T-shirts, three blue T-shirts, three white T-shirts but zero black T-shirts.

When you compare the three white T-shirts, question whether you *need* three white T-shirts, whether you wear all three, or if you can edit down to your most flattering and favorite two.

Maybe each T-shirt is noticeably different. One may be a long-sleeved V-neck, another a short-sleeved crew neck, and the third, a short-sleeved scoop neck.

Or they might all be short-sleeved crew necks. In this case, which is in the best condition, and which is the one that you always reach for?

While examining each piece, ask yourself whether you love it, sort of like it, or hate it. Go with your gut reaction. Don't agonize and overanalyze every single piece. Anything you look at and dislike can go.

Pieces that you take off every time you put them on can go.

If you look at something and find yourself wondering why you ever bought it in the first place, it can go.

Anything that's really looking worn or stretched can go.

And, of course, if you never wear it, it can go

Repeat this process with each clothing category. Continually remind yourself that you aren't going to let any emotional issues stop you from getting rid of clothes, shoes, and accessories that need to go. Keep your end goals for your closet and your wardrobe in mind.

Despite your newfound mindset, you'll still struggle to part with certain pieces. This is when you need to dig a little deeper to figure out why you're so determined to keep it when you never wear it.

Let's say you're looking at a red T-shirt. You really love the color, and you want to wear it but anytime you try, you take it right back off.

Why?

If you can't figure it out, you need to try it on and look closely at the details of the piece (as I just outlined above).

Additionally, ask yourself the following questions:

- Is it the fabric? Is it itchy, flimsy, or too hot?
- Does it end at part of your body that you prefer to camouflage and not call attention to?
- Is it an unflattering cut on you?
- Is it a beautiful color but not the best shade for you?
- Are you fussing with the sleeves, collar, or hem?
- Is it really your style?

Remember to use your utterly lame excuses list, fit check guides, clothing analysis flow chart, in-depth analysis questions, and wardrobe goals lists from your *An Imperfect Wardrobe Workbook which you can get at* https://closetcures.com/an-imperfect-wardrobe-workbook/ These will help you determine what needs to go and keep you moving.

If you're still struggling with whether to keep something after trying it on and conducting a thorough examination, the answer is right in front of you – it should go.

When in doubt, throw it out.

Bottom line: if you're not wearing it, no matter the reason, get it out of your closet. Once it's gone, you won't even miss it.

The Shelf

The top shelf in any closet is typically where heavy sweaters, sweatshirts, and off-season clothing are stored. But it can also be a place where pieces go and are quickly forgotten.

Unless you have everything in baskets or bins on the shelf, you'll have stacks that easily tumble over when provoked. This makes it annoying to try to get them out of the pile, which means you probably never wear these pieces. And if you're short like me you need a step stool to reach that high.

To tackle the shelf just remove one stack or bin at a time. Put like items together by category. Then, go through each piece while using your clothing analysis flow chart to help you decide whether it stays or goes.

Those of you with a closet organizational system may have a mix of hanging rods, shelves, and possibly drawers. If so, tackle one shelf at a time. Then, work on the drawers.

When you're done, neatly fold and stack all the things that you're keeping and return them to the shelf. Until you get the necessary storage pieces, like modular shelves, boxes, bins, and dividers, the upper shelf may still be stacked too high, but you can't just leave piles of clothes out.

The good news is you should have fewer items after your in-depth analysis. You may have also found some pieces that belong on the hanging rod or in drawers.

The Floor

Since most people keep their shoes on the closet floor, let's talk footwear.

Many women love shoes because your foot size rarely changes, and shoe sizes tend to be consistent from one brand to the next. This can make them more fun to shop for than tops and bottoms which can be emotionally draining. But it can also mean that you have more shoes than you wear.

Take out your shoes and group them by category such as sneakers, loafers, flats, heels, etc.

Go through each category one at a time asking the following questions:

- How many of each style do you have?
- Do you really need that many (maybe you do, maybe you don't)?

- Do you like them?
- Do you wear them?
- Are they still in good condition?
- Are they comfortable?

A good way to store the shoes you're keeping is to point the left shoe forward and turn the right shoe backward. This takes up less space. It also lets you see the front and back of each pair of shoes to help you when getting dressed.

Don't keep your shoes in the boxes they came in because you can't see what's inside. Instead, organize your shoes on shelves or in clear shoe bins. If you don't have modular shelves or shoe bins you can complete this task once you acquire the appropriate storage pieces.

Some of you may have categories other than shoes on the floor, especially if you already have some modular shelves, bins, and baskets in place.

If so, pull all these pieces out and evaluate whether they are staying or going. Determine if the keepers are staying on the floor or whether they belong with a category on the hanging rod or a shelf.

Dressers and Nightstands

If you have any clothes, shoes, or accessories in places other than your clothing closet, such as dressers, nightstands, or armoires, tackle those next. Use the same guidelines as above for deciding what stays and what goes.

A lot of people store their undergarments, socks, and bed clothes in drawers and dressers, so let's briefly discuss these two categories.

Undergarments include bras, panties, and any shape wear you may have. These are the foundation of your entire outfit; therefore, they should fit properly, provide the necessary support, and disappear under your clothes. Try each bra on to ensure it gives you the right lift, and that there is no spillage over the cups.

Socks are a category that never seems to get audited. Therefore, I'm willing to bet you have several pairs taking up valuable space that you never wear, that have holes, are thinning, or are missing their mates. Maybe they're in great condition, but you never wear them because they're too thick and make your feet sweat. Or maybe they're too thin and don't provide the best cushioning.

Sometimes they are just ugly!

Whatever the reason, if you don't like them and never wear them, just get rid of them.

Bed clothes are another neglected category that deserves attention. They are important because we spend a good chunk of each day lounging before bedtime and sleeping, so you need to be comfortable. Even if you live alone, you should still strive to wear bed clothes that fit properly and that you actually like. Use the same criteria for your bed clothes as for all the other categories.

Finally, let's tackle accessories, which includes jewelry, scarves, handbags, hats, and gloves.

Some people store their jewelry in decorative boxes on top of their dresser. Others store their accessories in drawers in their closet, or they use a hanging jewelry organizer. Although jewelry doesn't take up as much space as shoes, handbags, and clothes, that's no reason to continue to hold onto pieces that you never wear.

As you know, there's a difference between real jewelry and costume jewelry.

Real jewelry often comes with sentimental attachments because the pieces were family heirlooms, gifts, or something you purchased for yourself to celebrate an achievement. It also comes with a higher price tag. Therefore, it's understandable if you're struggling with whether or not you should part with real jewelry pieces you don't wear.

If it's sentimental, store it in your keepsake box.

If you suspect it has some value, remove it from your closet and consider selling it. This is the one category where it makes sense to take the time to try to get some money for unworn pieces. Alternatively, you can take it to a place that gives you cash for gold and silver. Costume jewelry, on the other hand, is relatively inexpensive. And it goes in and out of fashion faster than real jewelry. Evaluate each piece and be brutally honest about whether you like it and wear it.

Another category of accessories that many women own are fashion scarves and cold weather scarves. As with jewelry, scarves don't take up that much space, so it can be tempting to just keep them all. But that's not in your best interests.

Since a scarf sits right by your face, having only your best shades is the ultimate test of whether to keep it. If the scarf is not in your best shade, you probably don't wear it, and it should go.

The other element that impacts whether you wear a scarf is the fabric. Fashion scarves come in all fabrics, but do you really want a polyester scarf? Or one that's scratchy against your skin?

Scarves can be stored in baskets or bins, or you can hang them on hooks or hangers.

Gloves are like socks. If they have holes, are thinning, or you just don't like them out they go. And obviously, if one is missing, get rid of the other one.

Although you might store your handbags in the closet on shelves, we'll include them here with the accessory category. Many women use just one main handbag for the season or an entire year, and then they update it with a new one. But they still hang on to the old bag instead of getting rid of it. Even the highest quality designer handbags will look worn when used daily. They should be analyzed for condition, function, style, and color. Only keep handbags that are in very good condition, that you use, that you like, and that are in the same color tones as the rest of your wardrobe.

Jacket and Coat Closet

Unless you live in a perennially warm climate, you'll have an assortment of jackets and coats that you likely keep in a separate closet. Jackets and coats can be especially challenging to audit and edit because they typically cost more than the rest of your clothes and are not as trendy. They also take up a lot of room in the closet, so it's important to get rid of the ones you don't wear and never really liked.

Use the same criteria as the other categories to determine whether a jacket or coat should stay or go. Evaluate the fit, style, length, fabric, and color. As you try each one on, make sure you're wearing what you would normally wear underneath, such as a bulky sweater under heavy winter coats. Hug yourself to see if it's pulling across the back, bend your elbows, and take note of the sleeve length and whether it covers your wrists. Check to see if the buttons are still there and if they are getting loose, and make sure zippers still function smoothly.

*****

Congratulations! You've Completed Your Wardrobe Audit And Edit

Going through your entire closet, dressers, nightstands, and any place else you may have had clothes stashed is a project. By now you should have a nice pile of things to get rid of and more room in your closet.

Gather up all the garbage bags filled with unworn pieces that you accumulated as you did your category batch analysis. Put them in your car to take to the donation center.

At this point, you should be feeling a sense of satisfaction and accomplishment. Getting rid of perfectly good clothes is hard, but necessary in the pursuit of curating your *imperfect* wardrobe.

As you adjust to your newly merchandised, colorized, streamlined, and organized closet, you won't ever want to revert to having a jumbled mess of a closet filled with unworn clothes. This gives you motivation to keep control of your wardrobe. Don't be upset if you kept more clothes than you thought you would or thought you should have.

Remember, purging is hard, emotional work. Celebrate the progress you made and remind yourself that you'll continue to audit and edit over time. Seasonal edits and ongoing maintenance will help you to continue to purge and refine your wardrobe.

Going forward, you'll find yourself looking a bit differently at the items you were on the fence about. Most likely, they will be the next to go. Once that initial doubt about a shirt, coat, or pair of pants creeps in you'll be ready to part with it down the road.

It may take a round or two of editing, but you'll get there. The more you do it, the easier it gets. Remember, this is an ongoing process because your wardrobe and your lifestyle needs change and evolve over time.

8

Analyze Your Closet Setup

Now that you've merchandised and streamlined your clothes, shoes, and accessories, we can reevaluate your closet setup. The objective is to figure out how to maximize your space, no matter how large or small it may be.

Determine what is and is not working when reviewing the following categories of your closet set up:

- hanging items
- folded items
- socks
- accessories
- handbags
- undergarments
- bed clothes
- outerwear
- off-season clothes

For example, you may have tons of hanging space but not enough shelves for folded sweaters and jeans. You may also require a better solution for storing your socks, scarfs, and accessories, such as baskets or bins.

If you have the money, I highly recommend that you install a modular organizational system. These systems ensure that you utilize every inch of your closet, making it much easier for you to get dressed each day. For those of you with more limited funds, or who rent, you can replicate an organizational system with stackable shelves, drawers, baskets, and bins. Make sure to measure the depth, width, and height of each area for which you'll be buying storage pieces.

Once you decide what you need, like more shelves and baskets, you can go shopping for those items at your local box store, a specialty container store, or online. Think about the style and color you want. For the most streamlined and cohesive look, get your storage pieces in the same color, such as all black, white, or gray.

Your hangers should all be the same type, either wooden or plastic, with a metal swivel hook. Bright, plastic, multi-colored hangers will compete with your clothes and add visual distractions. Plus, you can't swivel the top. This is important because your clothes should all be facing in the same direction. The swivel top makes putting away laundry much easier.

Here's a tip: When you purchase new clothing ask if you can keep the hangers. Most stores use the same black plastic hangers with a silver metal swivel hook. The stores have way too many and will gladly let you keep them. That's how I transitioned from wooden hangers, which are bulkier and take up more room, to all black swivel top hangers.

List of what I need to get my closet organized: (example)

1. matching hangers
2. plastic bins with lids to store and stack off-season clothes

3. modular stackable shelves for shoes

List of what I need to get my closet organized:

1. _____

2. _____

3. _____

Use the Closet Organizational Analysis Worksheet from your *An Imperfect Wardrobe Workbook at* https://closetcures.com/an-imp erfect-wardrobe-workbook/

9

Wardrobe Maintenance

Keeping your wardrobe streamlined and in working order requires maintenance, care and attention to ensure that it continues to suit your needs. The goal is to prevent your closet from ever getting stuffed and out of control again.

Maintenance entails keeping an eye on your wardrobe throughout the season by conducting mini evaluations. It is also critiquing both your outgoing and incoming clothes at the change of seasons. Maintenance conducted in the form of mini evaluations will be easier than the full-blown audit and edit that you just completed. You will have fewer clothes and will be more rigorous in your editing.

This is the opportunity to get rid of pieces you were on the fence about during your first audit and edit. Once you've lived with your pared down wardrobe for a while, you'll be more inclined to part with clothes, shoes, and accessories that you don't wear and that don't fit into your wardrobe plans.

You'll also want to be on the lookout for any gaps that need filled. We'll discuss making plans to fill those gaps in detail in Part 4.

Change Of Seasons

It's a common practice for anyone living in a four-season climate to put away the outgoing season's clothes, shoes, and accessories, and bring out the clothes, shoes, and accessories that will be needed for the incoming or current season. The change in weather is the perfect time to reevaluate how well your wardrobe served you over the past several months.

The outgoing season pieces will be put away, possibly on those upper shelves, not to be seen again until next year. So, you don't want to just shove everything into storage bins or boxes without first deciding if you really want to store it for next year. As you pull the outgoing seasons pieces from your closet focus on what you did and did not wear.

Things to analyze with the outgoing season include:

- Does it still fit?
- Did you wear it?
- Do you like it?
- Is it still in good condition?
- Is it still your personal style?
- Does it still work for your lifestyle needs?

As you're putting the incoming or current season's clothing front and center, you can ask questions like:

- Are there some clothes that you wear all the time and that you anticipate will wear out soon? Or that are starting to show their age?
- Did you get rid of a bunch of worn out tank tops last summer that need replaced for the upcoming season?
- Maybe your winter coat is not looking as fresh as it did at the end

of last winter and you want to replace it?

If you revisit an item and are not excited at the prospect of wearing it again, know it doesn't fit quite right, and you rarely, if ever, wore it last season, then it should go. Chances are good that you probably struggled with whether to let it go at the end of the season last year but still held onto it.

Mid-Season

The mid-season maintenance evaluation entails looking at how your wardrobe is functioning right now in the current season.

Things to pay attention to are identifying pieces that you wear, but that are looking worn and will need replaced, identifying needed updates, and making plans to incorporate new styles into your rotation.

Frequent mid-season evaluation sessions are important because your needs can change all the time, not just at the start or end of a season. You may move, get a new job, or take up a new hobby. You may also get restless or annoyed with your wardrobe...

Whatever the reason, it's good to keep up with things by doing the occasional mini audit and edit sessions.

As the season progresses, you may find you want or need some new additions that you hadn't thought of before or just did not need at the time.

Again, the process for these mini-wardrobe maintenance sessions is similar to your original batch category analysis, but they are much faster and easier than your initial analysis session.

Use your Lifestyle Clothing Needs Worksheets, Category Batch Analysis Worksheets, Seasonal Wardrobe Purchasing Planner Worksheet and Your Warm and Cold Weather Seasonal Updates Worksheets to identify any wardrobe gaps.

Consult your **Wardrobe Analysis Flow Chart** to help you decide whether something should stay or go. **Get your free workbook at https://closetcures.com/an-imperfect-wardrobe-workbook/**

Wardrobe Audit and Edit Summary

Great work!

You've just completed the most difficult part of the process. It's not easy getting rid of your unworn clothes, shoes, and accessories, but now you can embrace the benefits.

You've streamlined your wardrobe so you don't have to fight with your stuffed closet when getting dressed. And you no longer have to see all your bad purchases every time you open your closet doors.

Your clothes are arranged by category and color. Not only is this very pleasing to the eye, but you also know right where to find everything.

And you know that everything fits properly, is in your best shade, is in keeping with your personal style, and works for your lifestyle.

You've also addressed any problems with your closet setup and have created a plan to get those systems functioning better.

Did you get rid of absolutely everything that you never wear?

Probably not. And that's okay.

In fact, it's perfectly normal for an *imperfect* wardrobe.

Over time, you'll fine-tune your personal style preferences, making it easier to purge. Pieces that you were on the fence about in your initial audit and edit session will likely be the next to go.

As I keep mentioning, getting the wardrobe you want is an ongoing process. It takes time.

In the next section, we'll figure out why you're buying the wrong clothes in the first place and what to do about it.

III

WHY YOU BUY CLOTHES YOU NEVER WEAR

Now we're going to shift the focus to figuring out why you buy clothes you never wear. Because that's where it all begins. The reason why your closet was so stuffed in the first place is a direct result of your shopping habits. Everything you buy ends up in that closet and contributes to how well, or how poorly, your wardrobe functions.

So, how can you ensure that you are making the smartest choices?

By being aware of your mindset. Just as your mindset impacts your ability to part with clothes, it also plays a role in your shopping trips.

We'll see how utterly lame excuses cause you to buy clothes you don't need.

We'll investigate how retailers use various tricks and tactics to entice you to make purchases, and how shopping at the wrong stores contributes to bad purchases.

We'll delve into how ignoring the big picture and the real cost of your clothes is hurting your wardrobe.

Finally, we'll see why shopping without a strategy is a recipe for wardrobe disaster. Download your free An Imperfect Wardrobe Workbook at https://closetcures.com/an-imperfect-wardrobe-workbook/

10

What Are You Doing Wrong?

You loved it at the store, but then you get home and ask yourself:
"What in the world was I thinking?"
"Why did I waste my hard-earned money on this?"
"Why am I buying all these clothes I never wear?"
"And why do I keep repeating the same process over and over again?"

There are six reasons why you have a closet full of clothes that you bought but don't really like and never wear.

1. Utterly Lame Excuses For Buying Something
2. Retailer's Tricks and Tactics
3. Shopping At The Wrong Stores
4. Ignoring The Big Picture
5. Unaware Of The Real Cost Of Your Clothes
6. Shopping Without A Strategy

Put all six reasons together, and they are a recipe for disaster in your closet. But once you are aware of these issues you will be empowered to make smarter decisions when shopping. Let's dig a little deeper.

11

Utterly Lame Excuses For Buying Something

Just as mindset plays a role in preventing you from getting rid of clothes you never wear; it also influences your purchasing decisions.

Shopping is like a drug. Many people get a high from the excitement of the mall, all the new arrivals and colors, and the seemingly endless sea of sale signs. All rationale goes out the window.

When you know you don't need something, but you want it, you try to justify the purchase by making utterly lame excuses.

Below are some common excuses we tell ourselves for buying something and why they are not valid reasons to pull out your wallet.

Utterly lame excuse for buying something...low price

Rationale: *I have this coupon and must spend "X" amount of money to save "X" amount. In fact, the only reason I came to this store today is to use the coupon I got in the mail, and it expires tomorrow!*

Reality: *You force yourself to buy something else to reach that goal. But you don't really like it, and you don't really need it, so you won't ever wear it.*

Price should be the final consideration, after establishing that it's a need, your style, and your best color. It should never be the only determining factor. Clothes, shoes, and accessories are worthless if you never wear them, no matter how good of a deal you thought you got.

Utterly lame excuse for buying something...that doesn't fit quite right

Rationale: *This jacket is so cool! It is a bit snug, but it's supposed to be formfitting.*

Reality: *So, you buy the jacket. But every time you try to wear it you take it off before leaving the house because you can't bend your arms.*

There's a difference between tight and formfitting. Trying to wear clothes that don't fit right only results in a long day of tugging at sleeves, fidgeting with waistbands, and just feeling off. If the clothes don't fit properly, leave them at the store.

Utterly lame excuse for buying something...I can always return it

Rationale: *I think this suit will work for me, but I'm not sure. I better get it just in case and I can always return it.*

Reality: *This one seems like a valid excuse. You certainly can return the suit. However, the problem is you typically don't return it. Or, you wait way too long and by then, you've lost the receipt, or you cut off the tags.*

If you're already thinking about returning something *before* you buy it, leave it at the store.

Utterly lame excuse for buying something...it looks good on someone else

Rationale: *Sara has this dress and I absolutely love it on her. She always looks so fashionable.*

Reality: *But Sara is six inches taller than you with the long legs of a model. And you really don't wear dresses.*

Never buy anything simply because you liked it on a co-worker, celebrity, or stranger. Only buy clothes that work for you.

Utterly lame excuse for buying something...to boost your mood

Rationale: *I'm so bored and depressed I think I'll go to the mall to see the new arrivals. I always feel better once I buy something.*

Reality: *Many people shop to lift their spirits, or because they're lonely or bored. This is also known as retail therapy. But it is bad because it's just a temporary fix. And once your mood shifts, that impulse purchase might not be as enticing.*

Find something to do besides shopping that does not involve spending your hard-earned money.

Utterly lame excuse for buying something...you did not come for

Rationale: *This raincoat is a beautiful shade of red and I don't have this color. I can buy the shoes I came for next time.*

Reality: *The red is much brighter than the reds you normally wear. And it's not a flattering shade for your skin tone and hair color.*

If it's not the right shade for you and if you really don't need it, then you're just wasting money and cluttering up your closet. Decide what you'll look for and stick to it.

Utterly lame excuse for buying something...it was on a must-have list

Rationale: *I need to get a white button-up blouse because it's on every must-have list I see.*

Reality: *But you don't like blouses because they gap at the chest and white tends to wash you out.*

One-size-fits-all must-have lists are a recipe for disaster. Everyone has different lifestyles, careers, wants and needs. Unless it's on your personalized wants and needs list, leave it at the store. This is not a must-have for you.

Utterly lame excuse for buying something...your fantasy life
Rationale: *This fun, sexy dress would be great to wear out to a nightclub at the beach.*

Reality: *But you're self-conscious in body-hugging clothes, haven't been to a nightclub in years, and don't have any beach vacations planned.*
Only buy clothes for your current, actual life that suit your lifestyle and personal preferences.

Utterly lame excuse for buying something...a friend or relative tells you it looks great
Rationale: *I'm going shopping with the girls on Saturday. It's always a good time trying on clothes and catching up on gossip at the same time.*
Reality: *Shopping with others can be fun. But your friends often have a different style than you.*

Don't let a friend or relative inject their likes and dislikes into your purchasing decisions. They don't really know what you need and often are not the best judge of what will work for you. Shop alone for serious buying trips.

*****

When you find yourself making utterly lame excuses to justify a purchase, it's a clear sign that you need to leave it at the store.

To curate your *imperfect* wardrobe, shift your mindset and focus on the wants and needs that you came in for.

12

Retailer's Tricks & Tactics

Retailers play a huge role in influencing consumer purchasing. They study ways to get people to buy things and they know all about the utterly lame excuses you use to justify purchases.

Companies also know that we make decisions due to being influenced by the way, or context in which, something is presented to us. This is called **behavioral economics.** Retailers use this information to their advantage because their main concern is their bottom line, not whether you need something, whether it fits right, or whether it looks good on you.

So they confuse and disorient you with the **store layout...**

They overwhelm you with way **too many choices...**

And they lure you with signs advertising **low prices...**

Store Layout

Retailers plan their floor layouts very carefully to entice you to go where they want you to go. There are rarely straight lines throughout the store. Instead, they make you weave in and out between racks and display tables.

Ever wonder why the fitting rooms, clearance sections, and checkout counters are located at the back of the store?

They know that if you're on your way to try something on you'll have to pass the clearance section. From there, you'll be compelled to check it out and, they hope, pick up a few more random pieces.

If you're returning a purchase, retailer's hope you will buy something else while you're in the store. That's why the cashier is located at the back. You must pass colorful, eye-catching displays designed to make you stop and, again, find some new pieces to purchase. Plus, that enticing clearance section is right there too. And at those checkout counters are where they strategically place small, inexpensive impulse items to tempt the shopper.

Don't let confusing store layouts distract you from focusing on what you came for. Get the pieces you want to try on because they're on your needs list and head straight for the fitting rooms. And if you're there to return something, head straight for the cashier and don't pick up anything along the way.

Way Too Many Choices

At first, having lots of choices seems like a good thing.

But remember earlier when we talked about how more choices can cause more problems?

There are so many places to shop and so many options in these stores, it's overwhelming.

Should you go to a traditional mall, the outlets, or a strip mall with big box stores?

If you choose the traditional mall or outlets, you're then faced with more choices. Do you want to go into every store or just the ones that catch your eye? And why are your two favorite stores located at opposite ends of the mall?

Once inside a store, you're faced with a ton of merchandise, pushy salespeople, and those enticing sale signs.

So, how do you combat the onslaught of choices?

Shopping with laser focus with purpose and a plan at the best stores for you. Stick to your list and your budget. Don't get distracted by shiny objects and sale signs.

Lure Of A Low Price

Retailers are aware that the lure of a low price can persuade even the most focused shoppers to buy clothes they had no intention of buying. Once you see those sale signs and tags with marked down prices, you get a rush of adrenaline. All logic goes out the window.

However, those low prices can be misleading.

While everyone loves a bargain, it often leads to buying things you don't need or even want. You end up with items that aren't flattering and don't fit in with your wardrobe in an attempt to save money on products you'll never wear.

The key before committing to a purchase is to ask yourself the following questions:

Did I set out to buy something like this today? If not, then leave it on the rack.

Do I need, or even want, this? If not, then leave it on the rack.

Is this something I'd be willing to pay full price for? If not, then leave it on the rack.

Would I even consider purchasing this if it wasn't on sale? If not, then leave it on the rack.

You also might wonder... why is this on sale? Why hasn't anyone else scooped this up? Is it because it's a weird color, a strange design, and a cheap fabric?

There's absolutely nothing wrong with buying something that's on sale if you need it. The same is true if it's appropriate for your lifestyle, your personal style, and is flattering on you. But if it does not meet all of these criteria, leave it on the rack.

Always remember, a bargain is no bargain if you never wear it. Instead, it just creates closet clutter, feelings of guilt, and is wasted money.

13

Shopping At The Wrong Stores

Your wardrobe is a combination of various items, bought at different locations and price points throughout the years. You buy a top here, a pair of pants there, and a jacket somewhere else. No wonder your closet can look like a cluster of unrelated clothes, shoes, and accessories.

Plus, if those pieces come from stores whose clothes don't suit your lifestyle, and don't work for your body type or your personal style, you won't wear them.

As I just mentioned, part of the challenge when clothes shopping is knowing which stores to visit because there are so many options.

The reality is that most stores simply won't work for your lifestyle, your body type, or your budget. This is part of the frustration many people experience when shopping. It leads to us blaming ourselves instead of the poor selection you find at the mall. While this sounds disheartening, it just means you need to do some legwork to find the best brands for you. It does take some time and effort to vet various stores. But it's worth it.

Retail companies have a specific client in mind when stocking their shelves. They design for a target age group and a certain lifestyle category. Each brand repeatedly uses fit models with the same body type and measurements. If you don't fit into their description, the store probably won't have much for you.

Therefore, you need to identify the stores that don't work for your lifestyle needs, that don't fit your body type, and that don't suit your personal preferences, and stop shopping there. You also need to identify the stores that consistently match your lifestyle needs, that fit your body type, and that suit your personal preferences. Once you do, shop these stores first.

Criteria To Determine If A Store Is Right For You

Store Windows and Mannequins: The mannequins give you a preview of what types of clothes the store sells. How are they dressed? Are they casual or more businesslike? Trendy or classic? Edgy or innocent? Are they appealing to you? Can you picture yourself wearing the outfits?

Atmosphere: What kind of music is playing? What age are the sales associates? How are they dressed? Can you easily walk around the store or is everything crammed together? Do you enjoy shopping there and could spend hours looking at every rack and table? Or are you anxious to escape?

Selection: Do you want to buy everything in the store? Do they have the pieces you need, in the colors you wear, and in the styles you prefer? Or do you struggle to find things you like?

Fit: Do most of the clothes fit well, or do they run too large or too small?

Price: Are most of the regularly priced items in your budget? Is everything on sale or just a select few pieces?

As you're searching for your best brands, you'll also learn which stores are not for you. **Knowing which stores to avoid is just as important as knowing which to visit**. Why waste your time and money in stores that never have anything for you?

If you're in a store and can't seem to find anything you like, nothing fits right when you do try something on, and it all seems too expensive, these are clues that you're in the wrong store.

Don't try to force yourself to like a store or an article of clothing. That's what leads to bad purchases and a closet full of clothes you never wear.

Think about the stores you visit the most and why you continually go there:

- Do you go there because it's convenient and close to home, or because it's your preferred choice?
- Do you buy a lot there, or do you do more aspirational browsing?
- Do you lose track of time while in the store? Could you stay there all day, or are you eager to escape?
- Do you like the clothes once you get them home? Are you excited to wear them, or do you question why you bought them?
- Do you wear them often? If so, do you really like how they look, or are they just okay?

Now think about the clothes you got rid of during your editing sessions. Do you remember where you got them?

If most of them came from the same handful of stores, then you should stop shopping there. Don't keep going back!

What about the clothes you kept? Where did they come from?

Once you pinpoint your best stores, spend most of your time shopping there and skip the ones that don't work for you.

Just as your wardrobe is an *imperfect* work in progress, so too will be your shopping trips. It takes time and effort to narrow down your best stores, but is necessary and well worth it.

14

Ignoring The Big Picture

When someone struggles with their wardrobe, it's usually because of a disconnect between what they like and need, and what they are buying. This happens when you're **ignoring the big picture.** The **big picture** is looking at your wardrobe as a whole entity rather than as lots of individual pieces. It is considering how the many different elements of clothes and shopping will work together. The colors, styles, and tone of the clothes, shoes, and accessories should be cohesive and compatible. Everything you buy should make a positive contribution to your wardrobe, instead of just taking up valuable space. And your purchases should be comprised of needs first and then wants.

You have an idea in your head of how you want to look or what you should be buying but it does not align with what you really want or need for your life.

You may want a sexy wardrobe for parties but spend most of your time taking the kids to soccer practice...

Or you may like how professional business clothes make you feel authoritative but you mostly work from home...

And you got everything on a must-have list you found online but you never wear any of it...

Ignoring the big picture leads to purchasing mistakes and a closet full of clothes you don't like and never wear.

Big-Picture Factors To Consider:

Where you purchase your clothes: This goes back to shopping at the stores that work best for you. The vibe of the store, the body type of the fit models, and their target customers remains consistent each season. When a good portion of your wardrobe comes from the same handful of stores the pieces should work well together.

While you don't want to be a walking billboard for a brand, sticking with stores that work for you will help you curate a cohesive wardrobe. Buying random pieces from various stores results in an incompatible mix of clothes, shoes, and accessories.

How will this new purchase will work with your existing wardrobe: Is it in keeping with the overall vibe of your wardrobe? Are the colors in the same tones? Do you have several pieces to wear with it? Do you know where you'll wear it?

Make sure any new purchases are in harmony with your existing clothes. Don't buy pieces that you'll likely only wear once, or that require you to buy additional pieces to make it work. That's focusing on the short-term and ignoring the big picture.

How will this new purchase work for your lifestyle: Are you buying clothes that you need or that you want?

If your closet is filled with lots of jeans and T-shirts but is sparse in the business casual department, you'll struggle to get dressed for work.

If you have a sexy wardrobe but spend most of your time carting kids around and running errands, you'll struggle to be appropriately dressed for daily activities.

And if you have lots of colors, prints, and patterns, but not too many neutral basics, then you'll struggle to put outfits together.

Instead, focus on finding pieces that work for the activities you do most often.

You should strive for a balanced wardrobe that has a mix of neutrals and pieces that pop, as well as clothes and price points in your best shades, in your style, and that suit your needs. We'll go into detail about these topics in the pre-shopping section of part 4.

15

Unaware Of The Real Cost Of Your Clothes

It was originally $80 and now it's marked down to $20. What a deal! I must have it...

I only need to spend $10 more to be able to use this coupon so let me find something else...

Buy 2 get 1 free. I only need one, but I might as well buy two and then I'll get a third one for free...

Have you ever found yourself saying something like this? I bet you have! I know I've used all of these reasons to justify purchases.

However, there's a problem with this rationale; it's not rational.

You think you're saving but unless you need it and will wear it, and wear it more than once, it's just a waste of money. A bargain is no bargain if it never leaves your closet.

Stop looking at how much *you think you're saving by buying* the piece and start looking at how much *you'd save by not buying* it.

Remember that you should never buy something based solely on the price. Instead, consider these four factors to determine the real cost of your clothes:

1. Cost-per-wear
2. Time spent earning the money
3. Enjoyment, confidence, and satisfaction
4. Entirety of your wardrobe

1. Cost-per-wear

To make the smartest purchases, estimate the cost-per-wear of each piece, not just the price listed on the tag.

What is the **cost per wear formula?** It's a method of estimating the true cost of a piece based on both the price tag and how many times you'll wear it. While not an exact science, it does help you make smarter decisions.

To figure out the cost-per-wear of individual items do the following:

Estimate the number of times you'll wear it per week and then multiply that by the number of weeks per year you expect to wear it. This gives you the estimated number of times you predict you'll wear it in one year. Then divide the cost by the estimated number of times per year you anticipate wearing it to get the cost per wear for one year.

Let's use a black leather jacket that cost $300 as an example.

Estimated number of wearings: 2 times per week x 30 weeks per year = 60 times per year

2 x 30 = 60

Cost of the leather jacket ($300) divided by the estimated times worn per year (60) gives you the cost per wear for one year ($5).

$300 / 60 = $5

How about one more example?

Perhaps you've been eyeing a bright patterned blazer that costs $75.

Number of wearings: 1 time per month x 6 months per year = 6 times per year.

So, take the cost ($75) and divide it by the number of times worn per year (6) to get the total cost per wear for one year ($12.50)

$75 / 6 = $12.50

The more expensive leather jacket is actually the better bargain because you estimate wearing it more often, thus making it less expensive in the long run.

You can even go one step further and estimate that you'll wear the leather jacket for the next 5 years, while the trendy, brightly patterned blazer will look dated after just one to two years.

Of course, these are estimates because you cannot predict with certainty how often or how long you'll wear a garment. But it does give you something to consider.

2. Time Spent Earning The Money

Another thing to consider is how long you had to work to buy that shirt, jacket, or pair of shoes. Unless you have unlimited funds, money is a factor.

If a sweater costs $60 and you make $15 per hour, you would have to work for 4 hours just to pay for it.

Is it worth it?

Maybe, maybe not...

It depends on your estimated cost-per-wear and how much enjoyment, confidence, and satisfaction wearing it will bring.

3. Enjoyment, Confidence, and Satisfaction

Picture something you have really wanted to buy but could not bring yourself to spend the money on like the aforementioned leather jacket.

Instead of spending $300 on something you really want and would wear all the time, you console yourself by buying a few T-shirts for a total of $60 even though you don't need any more T-shirts...

You also buy a pair of brown ankle boots that are marked down to $50...

And, while you're at it, you get another two pair of blue jeans on sale for $40 each...

By the time you leave the mall you have spent $190 on clothes and shoes that you did not intend on buying nor do you need. When you get home you're somewhat depressed because what you really wanted was that leather jacket. As you put away your new T-shirts next the extensive collection you already have, you can't help but think about that leather jacket and how much enjoyment you would feel every time you slipped it on.

Look at your purchases beyond the price tag. Flip the switch on your mindset and imagine the pleasure these pieces will bring you long after you forget the purchase price. You won't have the regret you'll feel when wearing something that you don't like but bought just because it was on sale.

4. The Entirety of Your Wardrobe

Have you ever thought about how much you spent over the years on clothes, shoes, and accessories?

Think about how much you spend each season and each year on your wardrobe.

Think about how much you spent on everything that's in your closet right now.

Think about how much you wasted on clothes you never wear.

Thousands and thousands of dollars were spent! So shouldn't you love and enjoy wearing everything that's in there? If not, you might as well have just tossed that money right out the window.

Start thinking of your closet as a whole entity, rather than as a random assortment of pieces. Look at it as a cohesive collection and as an investment.

Clothes are expensive, even when you buy them at a discount or on sale. When you spend a little here and a little there, you don't think about the entire cost. But it all adds up.

The purpose here is to make you aware of how much money you're spending on your clothes. Because whether you wear them or not, the money is gone. Even just a hundred dollars per month adds up to over a thousand dollars by the end of the year.

I'm not trying to make you feel bad or guilty, so don't get into that negative mindset. Instead, use this information to make better decisions going forward.

You must wear clothes so you should feel confident and comfortable in everything you own.

Therefore...*I want you to treat your closet like the major investment that it is.* Start thinking about your wardrobe as one large unit. This is the shift in thinking that will help you make smarter purchasing decisions.

Consider how new purchases will contribute to your existing wardrobe, how often you'll wear any new piece, and whether it will bring you enjoyment, confidence, and satisfaction.

16

Shopping Without a Strategy

Does this sound familiar?

You hit the mall excited about what new clothing you'll find. As you enter the first store you try to think about what you should look for:

A dress for that wedding in two months?

Maybe some new jeans?

More T-shirts in some new colors?

Without a plan, you wander around the store grabbing a few things as you go.

Before you know it, you have a hodgepodge grouping of items to try on including some dresses, jeans, and T-shirts.

Once you're in the fitting room you decide to start with the dresses. It's been so long since you even had on a dress that they all feel kind of strange. They're okay but you don't like any of them enough to commit to a purchase.

Next, you start trying on the jeans. But every pair you brought into the dressing room is either too baggy, too long, or won't even go past your thighs.

You're thinking, "When did they start having so many different cuts, styles, and lengths of blue jeans? How will I ever find the right pair?"

By now you're frustrated so you reach for your old standbys, the T-shirts. After trying on the rather large stack, you narrow your choices down to three. You already have a lot of T-shirts, but none in these colors. And you must buy something, right?

This is shopping without a strategy.

And this is what leads to a closet full of clothes you don't like and never wear.

So, what does shopping with a strategy look like?

It means you did pre-planning before hitting the stores. You thought about what you needed, how much you could spend, and where you were most likely to find those pieces.

Pre-planning is the best way to shield yourself from retailer's tricks and tactics, as well as to overcome the excuses that you tell yourself to justify your purchases.

Why You Buy Clothes You Never Wear Summary

Now you are aware of how your mindset impacts your purchasing decisions and leads to a closet full of clothes that you don't like and don't wear, as well as a drained bank account. Being aware of the utterly lame excuses you use for buying clothes, and retailer's tricks and tactics to get you to spend your money will help you make smarter decisions. Remember to shop in the best stores for you, keep the big picture in mind, estimate the real cost of your clothes, and shop with a strategy for the best results.

Perhaps you're thinking that this is a lot of analysis and thought just to buy clothes, shoes, and accessories. But, if you don't shift your mindset and shop more thoughtfully, you'll continue to make purchasing mistakes, waste money, and clutter your closet.

Once you get into a positive and purposeful mindset, it will be automatic. You'll be thinking about these things without even realizing it.

It's time to dive into shopping strategies that will help you have more successful shopping trips. In the final section we'll discuss pre-shopping preparation, the shopping trip, and post-shopping evaluation.

IV

SHOPPING STRATEGIES

*There are three key components to shopping smarter:
Pre-Planning, Shopping Strategies and Post-Shopping
Evaluations.*

*Before you head out to the stores, you need to think about
what you have, what you want, and what you need. You'll
use this information to create your wants and needs list,
which will keep you focused while shopping. The goal is to
look for pieces that will contribute to a balanced and versatile
wardrobe that consists of a mix of pieces in your most
flattering shades and in your personal style. These elements
make up your capsule wardrobe or personal uniform.
During the shopping trip, you'll decide what to look for, how
much to spend, where you'll go, and when to shop. You'll
learn the three P's of purchasing, and risks to be aware of
when shopping. You'll get tips and guidelines, along with
advice on fitting room checks and for shopping online.
Finally, you'll learn why it is so important to reexamine your
purchases once you get home to see how well they work with
your existing wardrobe. Once again, you can download your
free An Imperfect Wardrobe Workbook at
https://closetcures.com/an-imperfect-wardrobe-workbook/*

17

Pre-Shopping Preparation

Now that you have your closet streamlined, you're probably noticing gaps in some categories and a lot of very similar pieces in other categories.

Do not panic and think, "I should have kept all those clothes I got rid of!"

You were not wearing those clothes and having them in your closet did not help you when getting dressed. They only added more stress and confusion.

Instead, when going forward you should focus on curating an *imperfect* wardrobe better suited to your likes and needs. To do this, you must make smarter choices when shopping.

And how will you make smarter choices?

By planning *before* you go shopping.

Planning is done *before* stepping foot in any stores because once inside, you're susceptible to the overwhelm and retailer tactics we previously discussed. Even those with the best of intentions are vulnerable.

Just like we did mental prep work before tackling your closet edit, you must prepare before a shopping trip. Going clothes shopping without a plan is like going grocery shopping without a list: everything looks good, you forget what you have at home, and you forget what you need to buy.

Your goal is to have a wardrobe filled with clothes, shoes, and accessories that work for your daily lifestyle needs. To achieve this goal you have to determine what these needs are, what types of clothes will fulfill these needs, what you have, and what is missing. Then you'll create a list to guide you on your shopping trip to acquire these missing pieces.

But planning is more than just writing down that you need some new tops for work and a new pair of shoes for errands.

Since most of us cannot afford to buy everything we need and want all at once, you'll have to spread out your purchases. You must determine what you need, prioritize your most immediate needs, determine how much you're willing to spend, and think about where you're likely to find these pieces.

It's about looking for clothes that will bring balance, versatility, and cohesion to your wardrobe. These pieces should also be in your signature style and your best shades.

Before we dive into the best practices for creating your wants and needs list, let's discuss some key wardrobe factors that will help you create that balance, versatility, and cohesion.

18

Keys To Curating Your Wardrobe

The goal is to create a **balanced** and **versatile** wardrobe with the appropriate clothes for your daily activities. It should consist of **a mix of investment pieces, wardrobe workhorses, and fashion pieces** that are compatible because they are in the same color tones. These color tones should be **your most flattering shades**.

For maximum versatility, aim for lightweight pieces that can be layered or worn alone, and that are current but not trendy. Make sure your selections are in keeping with you **personal style preferences**. This is often called a **capsule wardrobe**, but it can also be called your **personal uniform**.

Now, let's break all that down!

1. What is a balanced wardrobe?

Balance is about the total number of pieces you have, and the proportion of pieces you have in each category and for each activity. Therefore, **a balanced wardrobe** will have an adequate number of pieces for each category of clothing and for each activity thus enabling you to easily get dressed.

An **off-balance wardrobe** happens when you have too much of one category, like casual wear, and not enough of another, like work wear. It can also occur when you have too many tops and not enough bottoms, or vice-versa. Having an off-balance wardrobe will cause you to struggle to get dressed.

An example of a balanced casual wardrobe:

- several T-shirts with different necklines and sleeve lengths in muted tones and neutral shades
- three lightweight cotton jackets with hems that end at different points, such as at the waist, below the waist, and at hip length, in those same muted tones and neutral shades
- an assortment of zip-up and pull-over sweatshirts in muted and neutral tones
- jeans in a few different cuts, like relaxed and slim fit, and different colors, such as dark blue, black, and gray.
- a few chinos in muted and neutral shades
- shoes include two pair of slip-on sneakers, one pair of slip-on canvas shoes, and one pair of loafers in muted and neutral tones.

An example of an off-balance casual wardrobe:

- lots of crew neck T-shirts in a mix of bright and muted colors
- three below waist, lightweight cotton jackets in bright blue, olive green, and red
- some pull-over sweatshirts in both bright and muted tones
- a few pairs of classic cut, medium tone blue jeans
- shoes include three pair of sneakers: one pair in bright green, one pair in purple, and one pair in a mix of bright colors.

Do you see why the first wardrobe is balanced and the second wardrobe is off-balance?

The first casual wardrobe sticks with the same muted tones and neutrals, the same types of garments, and the same cuts and silhouettes. This means every piece is cohesive and interchangeable, making it easy to get dressed. Interest is created with different necklines, different jacket lengths, and different types of bottoms.

The second casual wardrobe is not consistent with the color tones, all the T-shirts are crew neck, and the bottom options are limited to medium tone blue jeans. It lacks cohesion and has limited versatility making it difficult to create outfits that work together. Getting dressed is a struggle.

How does a wardrobe get off balance?

It can happen when you enjoy buying clothes for a hobby, but don't like buying more formal clothes for work...

You may also have trouble finding pants that fit, so you avoid shopping for them. This then results in only having one or two pairs that actually fit and are appropriate...

And you shop without a plan.

To correct an unbalanced wardrobe, you need to determine your best shades, and figure out your favorite and most flattering cuts and silhouettes. You also need to identify the duplicates and pinpoint the gaps in your closet. Then, you can make plans to create balance with your wants and needs list.

2. What is a versatile wardrobe?

A versatile wardrobe has many uses or applications. Individual pieces can be dressed up or down depending on what you pair it with.

Factors that contribute to the versatility include fabric, cut, and color. The most versatile pieces are usually neutral shades, solids or very subtle classic prints, and classic cuts and silhouettes, in all season fabrics. However, there are exceptions.

For example, a floral print, silk camisole can be incredibly versatile if the florals are in shades that work for you and with the rest of your clothes. If the flowers have bright green leaves and bold purple blooms with a vibrant yellow background, you can draw from any of those shades, provided the majority of your wardrobe is made up of bright, bold shades. The floral shirt can be worn alone, or you can add a cardigan or blazer that picks up one of the colors in the flowers. Another option is to pair it with a cardigan or blazer in a neutral shade of brown or white.

If versatility is the goal, having too many pieces that are only appropriate for specific situations or occasions creates a problem.

Here is an example:

Versatile: An A-line solid black silk sheath dress. It can be worn for work, a wedding, or church.

Not as versatile: A floral print, silk sundress with spaghetti straps. It cannot be worn to work, might be worn to a casual luncheon, but is probably not appropriate for church.

This drastically limits the number of times you'll wear the sundress.

How about another example:

Versatile: Black blue jeans. They can be dressed up with heels, a gold or silver belt, a silk camisole, and a lightweight blazer. They can also be dressed down with a concert T-shirt, leather jacket, studded belt, and boots.

Not as versatile: Army green cargo pants. They only work for casual activities due to the color and style. If you were to wear them with heels and a silk camisole, the outfit would not look right.

Of course, this is not to say you shouldn't have a floral print, silk sundress with spaghetti straps or army green cargo pants. If you really love them and will wear them a decent number of times, then add them to your wardrobe. Just limit the number of pieces that are not as versatile to get the maximum mileage out of your clothes.

3. What is a wardrobe mix?

A **wardrobe mix** is the percentage of price points, solids and prints, and classic and current styles that you have in your wardrobe. For maximum versatility and function, aim for a mix of approximately 20 percent investment pieces, 70 percent wardrobe workhorses, and 10 percent fashion pieces.

Investment Pieces | Best Quality | Long Term

Clothes, shoes, and accessories in the investment category will get a lot of wear for many years to come. This category should make up about 20 percent of your wardrobe.

In general, durability and lasting style come with a higher price tag. But investment pieces are worth the extra cost because you'll have them for many years and will wear them often.

Categories like winter coats, boots, designer handbags, wool and cashmere sweaters, and a well-tailored suit are good examples of investment pieces. The style and color should be on the neutral side since they'll be getting a lot of wear. However, some of you may want a signature statement piece like a bold green winter coat or a bright blue handbag.

Wardrobe Workhorses | Good Quality | Medium Term

Wardrobe workhorses are a mix of staples and versatile pieces that you expect to wear frequently over the course of several seasons. This category should make up the bulk of your wardrobe at about 70 percent.

While you want good quality pieces, that does not necessarily mean that they must be designer or the most expensive. You can find wardrobe workhorses in a broad spectrum of price ranges.

When you find a brand and style that you love and know you'll wear all the time, stock up and buy several in your best shades. Categories like lightweight jackets and blazers, blue jeans and trousers, and T-shirts and blouses are typical wardrobe workhorses.

Fashion Pieces | Average Quality | Short Term

Fashion pieces are on the trendier or more unique side. They work for a season or two but tend to look dated quickly and you easily tire of them. This category should make up about 10 percent of your wardrobe.

Since you'll only have fashion pieces for a short period of time, you don't want to spend too much on them. Because they are less expensive, the quality is typically lower which means they start to look worn after wearing them just a few times.

Use inexpensive fashion pieces to inject some new life into your wardrobe. These will be clothes that feature the latest trends from the runways, the colors of the season, and the currently popular silhouettes.

4. What is a capsule wardrobe?

A capsule wardrobe is made up of clothes, shoes, and accessories that all work together. You can easily mix and match most of your pieces because they are in the **same color tones and intensities, have similar silhouettes** that work for your body, are **similar types of clothes**, and have **a similar style**.

The idea behind a capsule wardrobe is that it creates a solid foundation which you expand upon according to your personal style preferences.

Many people put a limit on the number of pieces a capsule wardrobe should have. However, I'm not a fan of counting your clothes. The number of clothes you choose to keep in your closet is not as important as whether you wear them all, and whether they are working for your needs.

Quality is more important than quantity.

Some people argue that a capsule wardrobe is too restrictive or boring. That's because the advice for creating a traditional capsule wardrobe talks about neutrals, solids, and basics. But neutrals, solids, and basics do no have to be the entirety of your wardrobe. If you love prints, color, and variety, they can absolutely be part of your foundation.

Another way to create interest is with patterns. Mix two or more patterns into your capsule. You can choose smaller patterns so they are not as noticeable and are more classic, or go for bolder, larger prints and patterns. Remember the floral print blouse? It was a foundation piece because the color tones were cohesive, and you can wear it with so many different things.

Keep in mind that there's a huge difference between a navy and white T-shirt with subtle, thin stripes, and a red and white T-shirt with bold, thick stripes. While both are considered classic colors and prints, the navy and white T-shirt is more subtle and not as memorable. The boldly stripped red and white T-shirt, on the other hand, will be more noticeable and memorable.

Let's look at a few more examples.

A paisley print can be classic if the colors are more neutral and the print smaller, as opposed to an oversized paisley print in shades of bright purple and yellow.

Animal prints are another category that can go either way depending on the size and type of the pattern. Certain animal prints are considered classics, like leopard or crocodile prints, while others are bolder and tend to trend in and out, such as snakeskin and giraffe prints.

You can also add interest and versatility to your core foundation pieces by choosing jackets that end at different parts of the body, varying collar styles and necklines, and having a mix of textures including leather, linen, silk, cotton, cashmere, and wool.

I encourage you to create your own definition of an *imperfect* capsule wardrobe. Only you can decide exactly how many pieces you want and need, and what types of clothes to include. Because forcing yourself to adapt to someone else's definition of what you should wear is a recipe for a closet full of clothes you never wear and don't like. And that's what we want to avoid!

With that said, there are some general guidelines to follow to get the most out of your capsule wardrobe.

Use your own best and favorite **colors**. If those are purple, orange, and yellow, then add in one or two neutrals, like white or navy, and that's your capsule. Two people could have a capsule wardrobe with purple, orange, and yellow, but one person's might be bright, bold shades, while the other person's capsule might contain muted, subdued shades.

Wear clothes with **silhouettes** that work best for your body shape. Select silhouettes that flatter your figure and camouflage those parts that are not your favorite. Take note of where hemlines end, whether clothes cling, slightly graze or fall away from the body, and the overall shape and outline the clothes create.

The **types of pieces** you wear depends on your lifestyle, and your likes and dislikes. One person may prefer T-shirts and camisoles, while another prefers button-up blouses and polo shirts.

Your **personal style** is how you put your colors, silhouettes, and types of pieces together. It's the way you express yourself through your clothes. Factors that define your personal style include fabric choices, the details of a garment, and the accessories you select, as well as your color palette, silhouettes and types of pieces you choose. **How you put it all together is your *imperfect* personal style.**

For those of you who work outside the home, especially if your job has a more formal or businesslike dress code, you may need two capsule wardrobes: one for work, and one for leisure and errands.

Below are some general examples to give you an idea of the types of pieces you might have in each capsule. Again, you'll have your capsule filled with pieces for your specific wants and needs.

A **casual capsule** could have:

- 1-2 pairs of jeans
- 1-2 pairs of chinos or khakis
- 4-10 T-shirts
- 2 shirt jackets
- 1-2 casual jackets
- 2-3 pairs of shoes such as a pair of sneakers, a pair of canvas slip-ons, and a pair of loafers
- fabrics might be cotton, denim, wool, linen, spandex, and blends
- the color palette might be black, white, pink, green, and purple
- the silhouettes might be tight and curve hugging, shorter hems on skirts and jackets, and lower necklines

A **work capsule** could have:

- 1 suit
- 2-3 pairs of trousers
- 2-3 skirts
- 1-2 dresses
- 2-3 blazers
- 4-10 camisoles, button-up shirts, and silk T-shirts
- 1-2 pairs of heels, 1-2 pairs of flats, and a pair of boots
- 1 coat
- fabrics might be cotton, silk, cashmere, lightweight wool, and blends
- the color palette might be navy, cream, red, and yellow

- the silhouettes might be slightly form-fitting, with skirt hems around the knee, and more conservative necklines

Additionally, you may have a **warm weather** and a **cold weather** version of each capsule depending on the climate where you live. The **warm weather capsule** might include short sleeves and sleeveless tops, shorts, skirts, and open toe shoes, in lightweight fabrics like linen and cotton, while the **cold weather capsule** might include long sleeves, turtlenecks, pants, coats and boots, in warmer fabrics like leather, suede, wool, and cashmere.

5. What is a personal uniform?

Another term that's frequently used is personal uniform. Your **personal uniform** is the type of clothing you wear most of the time. It's putting your unique stamp on your capsule wardrobe with your choices of colors, fabrics, types of clothes and cuts, the accessories you add, and how you combine everything. You can also call it **your signature style or your personal style.**

A capsule wardrobe and a personal uniform are very similar, and the terms are often used interchangeably. But the difference is in the details.

Your personal uniform builds off your capsule wardrobe.

Many of us have a personal uniform but don't realize it. But being aware of how your signature style forms your personal uniform makes getting dressed quicker, easier, and less stressful.

Whether you prefer the term personal uniform or signature style they both mean you frequently wear the same:

- silhouettes
- tones and shades
- styles

- brands and designers

For example, my uniform would be T-shirts, blue jeans, and slip-on sneakers or shoes. When it's cold, I add a zip up hoodie or a lightweight jacket. That's my uniform. And it makes up my casual capsule.

Your uniform may consist of button-up shirts, chinos, cardigans, and loafers...

Or dresses, blazers, and boots...

Some of you may have a uniform filled with pieces similar to mine, but I might have solid T-shirts, traditional classic cut light blue jeans, and solid sneakers, while you may have striped and printed T-shirts, black skinny jeans, and boldly printed sneakers.

Both uniforms have the same pieces or elements, but each has a different twist based on the individual's personal style.

Again, if you work outside the home, you may have two versions of personal uniforms: one for work, and one for leisure and errands.

Over time, you may adjust your uniform as your wants, needs, lifestyle, and preferences change.

Having a personal uniform or signature style also means there are pieces and styles that you would never wear, such as a form-fitting dress and heels, or skinny jeans, or anything clinging at the waist and hips, and no oversized scarves.

Perhaps you avoid anything fussy, overly feminine, or revealing...

Or you would never wear pastel or neon...

This goes back to knowing what you don't like. It is just as important as knowing what you do like. And it all goes back to personal style preferences.

6. What is your personal style?

Your **personal style** is based on the types of clothes you're drawn to, that you choose to wear, and how you wear them.

I have concluded that there are three main overall personal style categories and nine sub style types that fall within the main three. The nine style types can be combined in many different ways to create your own unique, imperfect style.

Defining your personal style is a topic that is too broad to discuss in depth in this book. You can find more information about personal style on my website: **Closetcures.com**. Below is a brief summary.

The three style categories are:

• **Laid-back:** Those in the **laid-back category** dress in an easy manner. They don't like to fuss with their clothes, and they don't like wearing anything too stuffy, nor do they wish to be the center of attention. The **style types** that fall under this umbrella are **boho chic, relaxed, and urban.**

• **Being appropriate:** The complete opposite is the **being appropriate category.** These **style types** can be defined as **preppy, classic and euro chic.** They dress more formally than the other categories no matter what they are doing.

• **Being the center of attention:** Those in the **being the center of attention category** enjoy the spotlight. This **style type** dresses to attract attention by being overtly **sexy, feminine, and dramatic.**

Keep in mind that most everyone is a combination of at least two or three styles. However, you'll be most drawn to one of the three style categories. The mix of style types that you like is what forms your personal style.

7. What are your most flattering colors?

Wearing clothes in shades that flatter you is the easiest way to look your best. But figuring out those shades can be difficult and confusing. Like personal style, defining your best shades is a topic that's too broad and specific for this book.

There are tons of websites, quizzes and books that you can check out that are devoted to helping people determine their most flattering colors. However, many of them get way too detailed, which in turn, becomes way too limiting.

In my opinion, *Color Me Beautiful* by Carole Jackson is the easiest. It's the original and is still going strong because it is both simple and accurate. Based on the 4 seasons you're either a Spring, Summer, Winter or Fall. All that means is that you will look best in the colors found in that season. To break things down one more notch your skin has either warm or cool tones.

Because Spring and Autumn are warm tones many people can wear colors from both seasons. The same goes for Summer and Winter which are cool tones.

If you want a little more of a breakdown, each season is as follows:

- **Spring:** Warm, yellow undertones; clear, bright and delicate shades
- **Autumn:** Warm, orange and gold undertones; strong shades
- **Summer:** Cool, blue undertones; soft, cool shades
- **Winter:** Cool, blue undertones; icy, vivid, and clear shades

While it's important to know which shades look best on you, don't get too crazy with it, especially at the beginning. Use it as a guide toward making better purchases in your most complementary shades. You can find a link to the *Color Me Beautiful* quiz on my website: **Closetcures.com.**

Keep in mind, as with everything else, knowing which colors are not as flattering is just as important as knowing which are. This knowledge helps you breeze past clothes that are not in your best shades.

Sticking with the same color tones and shades creates a more cohesive and versatile wardrobe. When all the pieces work together in terms of colors they are easily mixed.

19

Wants And Needs List

There's one more thing we need to go over before you start working on your shopping list: the difference between a want and a need.

A **want** is something you would like to have.

A **need** is something you require to fill in wardrobe gaps or to replace a piece that's looking worn or is damaged.

Needs are more important than wants and should take a higher priority in your planning process.

Can a want be a need?

Yes!

For instance, let's say you need a new handbag because your current bag is starting to look faded, and the strap is about to break. That's a need.

Meanwhile, you've been eyeing a Coach bag that's a bit pricey.

This would be a want and a need. The best of both worlds.

Unless you swap out handbags frequently, you'll be using the bag every day. Therefore, you want a quality piece that will withstand heavy use, as well as a bag you're proud to carry. When you factor in the cost-per-wear the Coach bag makes sense, and would be a smart purchase.

How about an example of when a want is not a need?

You fall in love with a magenta raincoat on a shopping trip, but you just bought a new navy raincoat last year, and it's still in great condition. Therefore, the magenta raincoat is a want not a need.

So, should you automatically forget about the magenta raincoat and write it off as a frivolous waste of money?

Not so fast...

If you wear your navy raincoat a lot, sometimes it makes sense to have another option in your closet. Perhaps the navy raincoat is for work and the magenta raincoat will be for leisure and errands.

There's nothing wrong with buying a few wants each season if they're in your budget and work with your existing wardrobe.

That doesn't mean you should go out and buy five new raincoats in various colors and patterns.

Don't go overboard. That's how a lot of people get into trouble with their budgets and end up with an overstuffed closet filled with clothes that don't work for their daily needs.

Pick and choose when it makes sense to purchase something.

Tips For Creating Your Wants And Needs List

Your wants and needs list is a detailed list of any clothes, shoes, or accessories that you would like to add to your wardrobe. **Your *An Imperfect Wardrobe Workbook* contains a Lifestyle Activities Wheel to help you evaluate how you spend your time. Get it here https://closetcures.com/an-imperfect-wardrobe-workbook/**

The goal is to have the size of each category of clothing in your closet correspond with the size of that category on your current lifestyle activities wheel. So, if your largest wedges are for work and lounging, then the bulk of your wardrobe should have clothes for these activities.

When your clothing needs are not in sync with what you have in your closet you end up with a wardrobe that's off balance causing you to struggle to get dressed for certain situations.

Use the weekly activities wheel to determine the urgency of the categories:

- **Need immediately:** wardrobe gaps that cause you to struggle to get dressed
- **Need but not urgent:** updates to add interest and variety
- **Good for now:** no new pieces at this time

When creating your wants and needs list, be specific about the colors and styles that you plan on looking for when shopping. Think beyond the basic question of what you need and go into detail. **For example, if you just write down that you need a new winter coat that brings up all kinds of questions like:**

- Is it for work or errands?
- Do you need a longer coat to cover your legs when wearing dresses to work, or a short hip length coat for quick trips to the store, or maybe you need both?
- Are you in the market for a neutral black, or do you want to add a pop of color with a bright red shade?
- What type of fabric and style are you looking for? A sleek wool coat or a casual puffer jacket?

Let's look at an another example of why it is so important to be specific when listing a want or need.

There are many types of lightweight jackets including trench coats, barn coats, denim jackets, and rain slickers. To ensure you're dressed appropriately for your lifestyle, and the various weather conditions, you may need:

A more formal jacket for work such as a trench coat...

A casual barn style jacket for running errands...

And a rain slicker for your morning jogs.

Many people don't think about specific needs until, well, the need arises, and you don't have the appropriate clothes. This is when you struggle to get dressed.

Note that being prepared for your current lifestyle needs is different than having every type of garment on hand for any activity that might ever present itself. Only buy clothes, shoes, and accessories for your current lifestyle.

To help you create your wants and needs list, use your Weekly Lifestyle Activities Wheel and Current Wardrobe Allotment Wheel, Lifestyle Clothing Needs Worksheet, Category Batch Analysis Worksheet, Seasonal Wardrobe Purchasing Planner Worksheets, and your Shopping Wants and Needs List which you can download from your free _An Imperfect Wardrobe Workbook_. Get it here https://closetcures.com/an-imperfect-wardrobe-wor kbook/

When you're deciding what pieces you need:

- Work on one lifestyle activity at a time.
- List all the pieces you want and need in that category. Be specific.
- Rank items in order of priority keeping in mind that needs come before wants.
- Estimate how much you plan on spending for each piece based on whether it's an investment piece, a wardrobe workhorse, or a fashion piece.

For instance, if your work wardrobe makes up the largest slice of your activities wheel and it also has the biggest gaps that should be the immediate focus. You would make a list of the needed work items, rank them by order of importance, and then plan on devoting a larger portion of your budget to these pieces.

As I mentioned before, to curate the most versatile wardrobe, think in terms of fabrics and styles that can be worn year-round. Of course, your entire wardrobe won't be all-season fabrics. You might want some heavy wool sweaters for winter and breezy linen for summer. A wardrobe that's made up of about 50 percent of pieces that can be worn all year will serve you well.

Planning also includes thinking about your budget. Most people have limited funds to devote to their wardrobes. That's why it's so important to be clear and specific about your wants and needs.

Let's go back to the Coach handbag example and the cost per wear formula. A handbag for daily use provides more of a return on your investment.

But, if you really love the special occasion bag you may decide to buy it anyway. Just keep in mind that if the special occasion bag is more for the life you wish you lived, and not the one you actually live, it might be best to leave it at the store.

You can also make an **avoid it list**. This is a list of your wardrobe weakness, like T-shirts, that you want to avoid because you have more than enough. It's also a list of the styles and cuts that you know don't work for you. Again, it's all too easy to get overwhelmed at the store and having an avoid it list will help you avoid mistakes.

Because shopping can be so overwhelming it's best to shop for just a few pieces per trip, or to stick with just one lifestyle category of clothes. Don't try to shop for a new pair of jeans and a sheath dress for work at the same time. They are different categories and in different parts of the store. This will create confusion and make your shopping trip more difficult. Stick with one type of garment or one category to stay focused.

Some people say you should shop for complete outfits. However, I believe just about everything you buy should work with just about everything you already own, so focusing on complete outfits isn't necessary. And what is an outfit anyway? It's just tops, bottoms, shoes, and accessories. Let's not make things more complicated than they need to be.

When setting your budget, keep in mind the **big picture, the cost-per-wear, your long-term goals, and your enjoyment and satisfaction.**

Figure out **how much you want to spend** on each category and on each trip. Think in terms of **investment pieces, wardrobe workhorses, and fashion pieces**.

And think about **where** you might procure these garments and how much they are likely to **cost**.

These are all elements that form your strategy for the shopping trip.

20

The Shopping Trip

Now that you've prepared your wants and needs list, as well as your avoid it list, you're ready to hit the stores. Before you head out, **decide what you're looking for, your budget for the day, and where you'll go.**

What You Will Look For

Make a shopping list for each individual trip to take to the stores. This is not your extensive master wants and needs list. Rather, it's a short list of what you plan to look for on this specific excursion.

Below are some examples of things to consider:

- What category are you shopping for: casual wear or work clothes?
- What are the specifics of your target pieces such as colors, styles, fabrics, sleeve length, and hem length?
- Are you shopping for a want or a need?

How Much Will You Spend

Set your budget for the day based on what you're buying, and whether you're looking for investment pieces, wardrobe workhorses, fashion pieces, or a combination.

Remember to estimate the cost per wear and think carefully before each purchase.

Some questions to ask include:

- Does this piece fit my style?
- Is it in my best shade?
- Will it work with my existing wardrobe colors?
- Is it well made?
- Is this a long-term item, wardrobe workhorse, or trendy piece?
- What do I like about it?
- Does it look good on me?
- Is it flattering or does it call attention to areas about which I am self-conscious?
- What is the fabric content and how does it feel next to my skin?
- Is it worth the price?
- Does it look in keeping with my existing personal uniform pieces?

Where Will You Go?

Most of us conduct the majority of our shopping trips at our local mall, and will occasionally visit a mall across town or in another city. If you're having trouble finding clothes you like, try visiting a different mall. The closer you live to a larger city, the more shopping options you'll have without traveling too far.

For instance, where I live in Pittsburgh, there's a large regional mall just miles from my house. However, the variety of stores is less than ideal, and it's looking dated and sad. (Fun fact: This is also the Monroeville Mall where they filmed the classic movie *Dawn of the Living Dead.* Funnily enough, this mall is now just about dead.)

But if I travel to the northern outskirts of Pittsburgh there is what is considered a "Class A" mall with more upscale stores. If I travel to the west, there's an outlet mall. There's also a "Class B" mall to the east. I'm fortunate to have several shopping options to choose from if I'm willing to drive an hour or two to get there.

While you may not always want to travel too far, the occasional excursion to a different mall can result in some great finds. You might even discover some new favorite stores that you weren't aware of. If you do come across some retailers that you like but that are a bit further from home, you can then shop them online with confidence.

Seek out the brands that fit you well and work for your lifestyle. It may take some time and effort but it's well worth it. Different stores have different target customers. Make sure you're shopping in stores that are age appropriate, that have the vibe you're going for, and whose clothes fit you well. As I mentioned before, brands use the same fit models to get consistent cuts, and each brand has it's own specifications. That's why a size 10 in one store will fit, but a size 10 in another store or another department may not. This can be frustrating. And this is why it takes time, trial, and effort to find your best brands.

Once you do find a few brands that work for you do the bulk of your shopping at their stores and on their websites. This saves time and eliminates buying mistakes. Sticking with the same brands also creates cohesion. A designer's collections tend to work together from one year to the next.

Let's compare two brands: Coach and Michael Kors. Both companies are upscale designer brands that are still within reach for the average consumer. However, each has a different vibe.

Coach is a classic, old-school brand that's more conservative with muted shades, while Michael Kors is trendy and vibrant with bright, bold shades. Both are high-quality, well-loved brands but some people may view Coach as too conservative, and others may view Michael Kors as too trendy.

When To Shop

Stores get new merchandise all the time. However, the types of clothes, shoes, and accessories that are in stock varies throughout the season.

Whether you're shopping online or in person, you'll find:

- a limited selection of pieces at full price at the start of each season
- the best selection and widest range of prices toward the middle of each season
- the worst selection and lowest prices at the end of each season

As a new season begins, like Spring, stores will still be trying to unload any leftover Winter merchandise. It's best to avoid shopping at these times if you're highly susceptible to the lure of low-priced clearance items.

However, the first few weeks of a new season is also when retailers start getting new arrivals. This is a great time to shop for those who like to get an early start on updating their Spring wardrobe. Pieces will be arriving slowly and the stores won't have their full stock of new Spring merchandise yet, so your options will be limited. You'll also be paying full price.

Just before the halfway point is when stores have the majority of the current season's new merchandise fully in stock. The prices might still be a bit high, but can be well worth the investment when it's something you really need or want. This is the best time to find the size you wear and the shades that flatter you.

If you wait for the price to go down, you risk the store being sold out of your size or preferred color. Plus, you need these pieces and want to wear them for the current season, so waiting for a sale is not always optimal. Use the cost per wear formula to help you decide whether it makes sense to commit to a purchase.

Fill in any wardrobe gaps with mini-shopping trips throughout the season. These occasional shopping trips are necessary because maybe there was something specific you wanted but could not find at the beginning of the season...

Sometimes a new need arises...

Or sometimes you simply decide you want something new.

Just make sure that anything you buy fulfills a want or need, is in your best shade, is in keeping with your style, and works with your budget.

Despite being an obvious statement, it bears repeating: Keep the receipts!

Although this is common knowledge, the problem is many people never return pieces they regret buying because returning clothes is a hassle. However, it is necessary if you suspect you won't wear it and don't want it cluttering up your closet.

When you get home and see your new purchases with the rest of your wardrobe they don't always work well together.

Perhaps you bought a dress for your fantasy life, but once you get home you snap back to your real life and know you'll never wear it.

Instead of returning it you cling to it in the hopes that one day you'll need it...

You might get invited to a fancy dinner party...

Or a last-minute weekend ski trip.

And the cycle of making utterly lame excuses for keeping clothes you never wear continues...

This is what we want to avoid. The entire purpose of this book is to guide you on the path to having a closet that is only filled with clothes, shoes, and accessories that you like, need, and wear. Because you don't need to get rid of unworn clothes if you never buy the wrong clothes in the first place.

*****

You did your pre-shopping preparation, thought about which stores you would visit, set your budget, and prepared your list. As you're shopping remember to stay focused on your end goals: to only spend your hard-earned money on clothes, shoes, and accessories that you need and that work for your lifestyle. They must be in keeping with your personal preferences, work well for your body, and be in your best shades. And you must stay within your budget.

An easy way to remain focused is to always keep in mind the **Three P's of Purchasing:**

1. **Planning:** Knowing what you need and want
2. **Psychological:** How you feel in the clothes
3. **Price:** Staying within your budget and using the cost-per-wear formula

Things To Be Aware Of When Shopping:

- Negative though patterns, emotions, and misleading mindsets – be aware and then flip the switch
- The lure of the low price – price should be the last consideration
- Confusing wants with needs – snap back to reality by reviewing your needs list
- Straying from your list - if you need blue jeans don't get sidetracked by the blazers.
- Making excuses to justify a purchase – only buy if it fits properly, is in keeping with your style, is in your budget, and is on your needs list

- Buying what you think you should buy instead of what you want to buy – stick to your own must-have list
- Analysis paralysis – if you can't decide then walk away, or buy both, but keep the receipts and vow to return one if you realize you don't need it or want it
- Sensory overload – take a break, have a snack, and a beverage
- Decision fatigue – know when it's time to call it a day

Shopping Tips and Guidelines:

Dress appropriately. Wear clothes that are easy to take off and put back on in the dressing room. Wear comfortable shoes. If you can, leave your coat in the car. Carry a light, small handbag, like a crossbody, so you don't have to fuss with it.

Avoid crowds. Shop early or mid-morning on a weekday when fewer people are shopping. The stores will be freshly merchandised from the night before, the floor will be stocked, and the checkout lines will be shorter.

Stick with your best brands. You know they work for your body and your budget. Plus, their clothes work together over several seasons. It also makes buying online easier.

Analyze quality, construction, and fabric. Really examine everything you're considering. Buy clothes for their features, not just a brand name.

Choose interchangeable pieces. Look for all-season pieces, in your best shades, that you can mix and match to create multiple looks.

Stay within your color palette. Don't be swayed by beautiful colors and fun patterns that are not in your best shades. Just because you like a color does not mean it will look good with your skin tone, hair color, and eyes. And it won't necessarily go with the rest of your wardrobe.

The Fitting Room

While shopping can be fun, there are times when you really should treat it almost as a job.

If you're in the market for a new pair of jeans go to your favorite store where you usually have success, or a large department store that has lots of options. Try on every cut that you're curious about or that has worked in the past. Don't bother with those styles you know you don't like, such as tapered legs or a high waist.

Sizes will vary from brand to brand, and from cut to cut. While you may fit comfortably into a size ten pair of Levi's, you might have to go up or down a size in other brands. That's why you have to spend time experimenting.

If you're unsure about the size and fit, especially if this is a new store for you, take a size up or down with you into the fitting room in addition to the size you think will work. Otherwise, you'll have to get dressed, trek back through the store, and retrieve another size, go back to the fitting room, and get undressed again.

It can help to take a few different colors, as well. However, fitting room lighting is notoriously bad so you might not get a true read. That being said, if you know which colors and shades look best on you and are in your color palette, you should be able to judge the color before you get to the fitting room.

Replicate Your Movements

When trying on any garment, you should replicate the movements you do throughout the day like sitting, bending over, walking, and lifting your arms. You can't truly judge the fit and feel of a garment by standing in one spot. If something is bothering you after just a few minutes, imagine how annoying it will be during a long day at work or while running errands.

Most retail fitting rooms are also tiny making it impossible to judge how pieces feel while you're in motion, therefore, you may want to leave the fitting room and walk around the store.

Although these are not ideal conditions for analyzing clothes, you must do the best you can. Once you learn what to look for regarding proper fit and what works for you, selecting flattering garments does get easier.

This will also help to ensure that you're going to love the piece and get the maximum usage out of it. The last thing you want to do is purchase something and never wear it.

Mirror Check

Pay attention to features such as where the shirt hem falls on your body, where the skirt or shorts end, and how low the neckline plunges. Close your eyes, then open them and see where you eye goes. Make sure your gaze is landing on a spot that's flattering and a part of the body you want to emphasize rather than conceal.

How Do You Feel In It

Take note of how the fabric feels against your skin. Avoid material that's scratchy and hot, buttons or zippers that dig into your skin, and waistbands that squeeze your stomach. You should feel comfortable and confident, instead of being distracted by what you're wearing. Again, if it doesn't feel right in the fitting room, the comfort level isn't going to get any better after you buy it.

Details Do Make A Difference

Beyond the comfort level and ensuring you don't bust a seam, you also need to pay attention to details such as pocket placement, design lines, buttons, zippers, and fabric weight. These seemingly minor details can greatly impact how an item will look and feel on you.

*****

Use these guidelines to make sure everything fits properly before spending your hard-earned money. Then you'll be shopping smarter so that you look better and love your wardrobe. Take the **List of Fit Checks from your *An Imperfect Wardrobe Workbook*** to help you decide whether to commit to a purchase.

Shopping Checklist

- Is this a want, a need or an impulse buy?
- Does it work for my lifestyle?
- Is this my best shade?
- Is it in my personal style?
- Does it have the vibe I'm going for?
- Does it fit?
- Is it comfortable?
- Is it flattering?
- Is it in my budget?
- Do I really like piece or just like the price?

Shopping Online

Follow the same guidelines for shopping online as you use for in-store shopping with a few additional caveats as outlined below.

Proceed with caution.

Since you can't feel the garments or try them on before buying, it's even more important to know your best brands, the fabrics you prefer, and the cuts you like when shopping online. If you've been to the brick-and-mortar store, you know how the clothes fit and the overall vibe of the brand.

If you do want to try a new company, but there's no brick-and-mortar store near you, start by buying just one or two pieces. See how they work out it terms of fit, fabric, and style.

Pay attention to the body type of the model.

The models wearing the clothes in the pictures used online are just that, models. They were selected because they look good in everything the company is trying to sell. If the model doesn't have the same body shape as you, then the picture is not an accurate representation of how the garment will look on you.

Many companies are using a larger variety of models with different figures. However, that model may still not represent you. That's why it's so important to be aware of which cuts, silhouettes, and colors consistently work for you.

Know your fabrics.

Different fabrics have different elements. The percentage of each fiber will contribute to the look, comfort level, and feel of a garment. Since you cannot try pieces on before buying online, it's important to know how different fabrics can impact fit and feel.

For example, a basic T-shirt made from synthetic fibers will cling to the body, can be hot, and will be thin. Whereas, a natural fabric, like cotton, will not cling, will not be hot, and is typically thicker thus providing more coverage.

Blends offer the best qualities of both natural and man-made fibers. Certain synthetics can reduce wrinkles and provide more shape. However, adding even just one or two percent of a synthetic fabric to a natural fiber can drastically impact the look and feel.

Factor shipping costs and possible return fees into your budget.

Many sites offer to let you "take advantage of their free shipping" provided you purchase a minimum dollar amount. This is one of the many tactics online retailers use to get you to buy more than you originally planned.

Isn't it funny how the one or two items you decide to buy always seems to fall just short of the required minimum amount? So, what do you do? You find something else to buy. This isn't necessarily bad if, again, you know the brand, the fit, and you can buy it in a second color. However, if you're making yourself buy something simply to qualify for the free shipping, you're just spending more money. It might be cheaper just to pay for that shipping!

Read the customer reviews.

The takeaway here is to judge the overall customer reviews for a company before deciding to order from them. What's the theme of the reviews: bad fit, poor quality, or a shipping issue? Several bad reviews for a piece may just be one bad item, but numerous bad reviews for most products should be a warning sign about the company. Steer clear!

21

Post-Shopping Evaluation

How many times have you returned home from a day of shopping and, upon looking at your newly acquired pieces, wondered what you were thinking?

These are not the pieces you went for.

They are not part of your color palette.

And you don't know where you're going to wear them.

But what happened?

You did your pre-shopping preparation, thought about which stores you would visit, set your budget, and went with laser focus to get the items on your needs list.

At the store, you were excited about the clothes because they seemed to fit your criteria. You thought you were making wise purchasing decision and you just had to have them.

But now that you're back home questions and doubt creep in...

Did I pay too much?

Do I really like it?

Do I even need it?

Will I ever wear it?

Do I really need one in every color?

If this sounds familiar, you're not alone.

We've all experienced it. The rush of buying something, and then the onslaught of guilt. It's called **buyer's remorse, or post-purchase guilt**.

Then, instead of returning the clothes, you rationalize your purchases because you can't admit you made a mistake. You justify your purchases by focusing on the positive attributes, like the color. But, you conveniently overlook the negative attributes, like the high price tag and slightly snug fit. This is **post-purchase rationalization, or choice-supportive cognitive bias**, which is how you end up with a packed closet full of clothes you never wear.

Months later, you find those items still hanging in your closet, yet to be worn, with the tags still on them long after the return period expired.

Unfortunately, we all make mistakes. And sometimes we simply fall victim to retailer's tactics and succumb to the rush of buying new clothes. After all, you're only human!

Don't berate yourself and give up. Acknowledge that this is perfectly okay and normal, and vow to do better next time.

Developing successful shopping strategies takes time and effort.

Refining your personal style involves trial and error.

And it takes commitment to the practice of mindfulness to ignore that inner voice whispering that you need that gorgeous purple jacket when you didn't come shopping for it.

This is why it is so important to reexamine and rethink your purchases when you get them home.

As you evaluate your new purchases, think about your thought process at the store.

- Were you thinking about your fantasy life and not your real life?
- Were you thinking about just in case situations?

- Did analysis paralysis cause you to buy too much out of fear of making the wrong decision?
- Were you ignoring the big picture?
- Did you forget about estimating the cost per wear because there was a buy two get one free sale?
- Were you shopping at a new store that you now realize may not be for you?

Look at your new clothes in the closet with your existing wardrobe.

- Do they seem like they belong? Do they blend in because they're very similar to what you already have, or do they stand out because the vibe is different?
- Do the colors work with your color palette? Are they the same tone and intensity? Or do they stand out because the color is off?
- Try them on and see how they look in normal and natural lighting. Combine them with some of your existing pieces to create new outfits. If you're having trouble pairing them with things it's a red flag. Remember, most pieces should work with the other pieces in your wardrobe.
- If your new purchases are replacements or updates for existing clothes, shoes, or accessories that were looking worn be sure to get those old pieces out of your closet and dispose of them.

Shopping Strategies Summary

How can you cut down or eliminate bad purchases and buyer's remorse? Prepare ahead of the trip by identifying what you need, what you'll look for, and how much you can spend.

Have a shopping plan and stick to it.

Be honest and listen to your gut. Recognize when you're making excuses for buying something. When you buy pieces based on utterly lame excuses, this quickly turns into post purchase guilt.

Reexamine your purchases once you get home. Don't cut off the tags or throw away the receipts until you evaluate the clothes, shoes, and accessories with your existing wardrobe, and not until you wear the them.

Acknowledge that you'll still make the occasional bad purchase. That's okay and perfectly normal. Simply return the items, learn from the situation, and vow to do better next time.

22

Conclusion

Congratulations!

That was a lot of introspection and hard work, but now you're well on your way toward curating an imperfect wardrobe that works for you.

At this point, you should only have clothes, shoes, and accessories in your closet that fit you properly, are in keeping with your personal style and lifestyle needs, and that you like and wear.

When you open your closet, you'll experience a feeling of calm because everything is color coordinated and organized by category.

As you get dressed, you'll easily find whatever you're looking for because it's not so overstuffed that you can barely even squeeze your hand between the garments. You know exactly what you have saving you time and aggravation getting dressed.

You created a new, positive mindset that will help you as you continue to shape and build your wardrobe.

The basic principles of auditing and editing will become a normal, unconscious habit for you. You'll easily maintain this new and improved closet without too much effort because it's streamlined, organized, and colorized.

Further, you've figured out why you were buying clothes you never wear. You won't justify purchases with lame excuses, and you won't let a retailer's distractions deter you from your shopping strategies.

You will only shop for the items on your wants and needs list while staying within your budget, and you won't settle for anything that does not fit your personal criteria.

You will go through your day without stressing about your clothes because you'll know you look your best, and you'll be comfortable because everything fits you properly.

Even though you'll still grow bored with your wardrobe every now and then...

You'll hold onto some pieces longer than you should...

And you'll continue to make the occasional buying mistake...

Don't let things like this discourage or deter you.

Remember that there is no such thing as a perfect wardrobe or a perfect person...and that's okay.

The best, most perfectly imperfect wardrobes evolve over time and improve with care and attention.

Give yourself permission to embrace your imperfect wardrobe!

V

Thank You For Reading

I hope this book has inspired you to reclaim control of your wardrobe.

I really appreciate your feedback, and I love hearing how An Imperfect Wardrobe has helped put you on the path to loving your clothes.

Could you leave me a review on Amazon letting me know what you thought of the book?

Thank you so much! You can find even more information on my website: https://www.closetcures.com.

VI

About the Author.

Linda is a wardrobe strategist and the creator of Closetcures.com where she helps women curate a wardrobe that works for them. She has a bachelor's degree in Fashion Merchandising, a master's in Asset and Property Management with a concentration on retail stores and shopping centers, and a certificate from The Image Maker, Inc program for image consultants. Linda reads every style and image book she can find. Through her many years of education, research, career, and personal experience, Linda has come to understand why we have so many clothes we never wear, and what we can do about it.

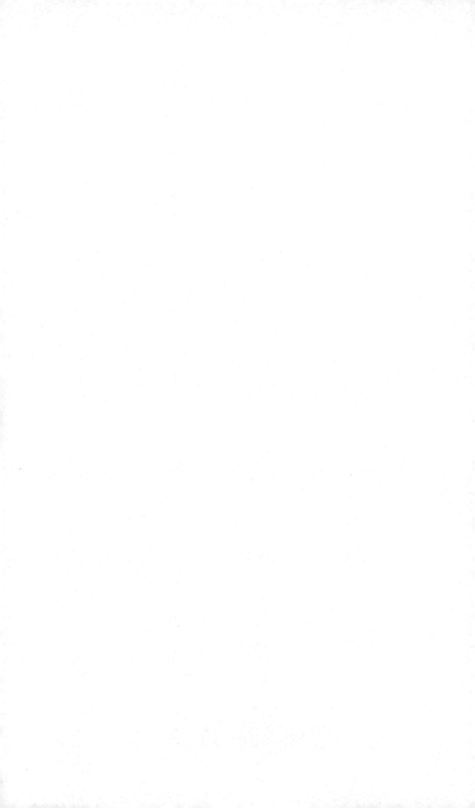

Made in the USA
Las Vegas, NV
21 October 2022